Contents

Introduction

A new scientific truth does not triumph by convincing its opponents...
but rather because its opponents eventually die,
and a new generation grows up that is familiar with it.

Max Planck (1949), German physicist, Nobel Prize winner

We all know somebody who suffers from heart disease or who has died from it, including members of our own families. Heart disease is our modern plague. We hear about it in the popular media, every time we see a doctor, every time we talk to friends and neighbours, and every time we buy our food. It has become a background noise for many of us, so we don't stop and think: what on earth is heart disease and should I be concerned about it?

People may suffer from many different heart problems, such as rheumatic fever, congenital heart defects, infections, tumours, heart muscle disorders, injury, damage from drugs and other toxins, genetic disorders, and heart failure. However, when people talk about "heart disease", what they mean is *Coronary Heart Disease (CHD)*. Why? Because it is the number one killer in the Western world: more than a third of people in developed countries die from *CHD*.[1,2] Despite the fact that the death rate from *CHD* has reduced somewhat in the last 15 years, the number of people falling prey to the disease is still growing.[2] And yet at the beginning of the 20th century *CHD* was so rare that it was not described in major medical textbooks because doctors virtually never saw it. Today an estimated 17 million people around the world die from cardio-vascular disease every year and the most rapid growth is in the developing countries where heart disease is gaining epidemic proportions.[2,3]

CHD is thought to be caused by *atherosclerosis*

What is atherosclerosis? It is a disease of the arterial wall that leads to narrowing and obstruction of the artery. The narrowing is due to the sclerotic deformation of the artery and the development of raised patches, called atherosclerotic plaques, in the inner lining of the arterial wall.[4] Depending on which organ in the body the artery feeds, atherosclerosis in its walls will impair the blood flow to that organ.

Let us have a look at the organs that are most affected.

1. Atherosclerosis of the arteries feeding the heart (called coronary arteries) results in our most common cause of death – *Coronary Heart Disease (CHD)* – the disease this book is about.[1]
2. Atherosclerotic damage to the arteries feeding the brain causes *strokes* – our third most common cause of death (after cancer).[2]
3. Atherosclerosis of peripheral arteries causes *Peripheral Vascular Disease* with symptoms of painful muscles, cold extremities, ulcers and gangrene.[4]
4. Atherosclerotic damage to kidney arteries can lead to high blood pressure and kidney failure.[4]
5. Atherosclerosis of intestinal arteries can lead to severe abdominal pains and digestive abnormalities; it may also result in gangrene of the intestines.[4]

Wherever atherosclerosis develops it impairs blood flow, and hence the function of the organs and tissues fed by that artery.

The two major forms of *Coronary Heart Disease (CHD)* are *angina pectoris* and *myocardial infarction* (heart attack).

Angina pectoris develops when the lumen (the space inside) of the coronary artery is narrowed, but not closed up. So, when a person is resting the heart can cope with the lowered blood supply. But when the person does some physical activity and the heart muscle has to work harder, the atherosclerotic artery cannot supply enough blood to feed the heart muscle. The result is a very typical gripping chest pain behind the sternum, usually radiating to the neck and left arm, rarely the right arm. The pain disappears with rest in the initial stages. As the disease progresses the person has to take medication (glyceryl trinitrate or other nitrate drugs), which dilates the artery and improves the blood flow, so the pain stops.[5]

Heart attack, or myocardial infarction, happens when the coronary artery closes up completely and the blood supply to the heart muscle stops. The result is the death of the portion of the heart fed by that particular artery.[5] It can happen in a person who has never had any heart symptoms, or in a person who has suffered from angina for years. Typically the heart attack is manifested by severe chest pain that is not connected with any physical activity and not helped by nitrates. The pain is usually accompanied by extreme fear, cold sweat, nausea and shock. In rare cases heart attack may be silent, without the pain. About half of all people who have a heart attack die in the first 2–3 hours. Those who make it through the first few hours take weeks to recover. They are left with a scar in the heart muscle, which may lead to arrhythmia, heart failure and other complications. *Arrhythmia* is an abnormality in heartbeat caused by a disturbance in the electrical conduction system of the heart. Both angina and infarction can lead to arrhythmia.[4,5]

Modern medicine has developed an arsenal of means to help us survive *Coronary Heart Disease*: various drugs, artery bypass surgery, balloon angioplasty and even heart transplant. As a result the death rate from heart disease has decreased somewhat in the last 15 years.[1,2] However, medicine has no cure to offer you. So, once you have *CHD* you may need medical help for the rest of your life. Therefore the real question is: how do we prevent heart disease? In order to understand that we need to know how to avoid falling prey to the real modern plague – atherosclerosis.

Atherosclerosis has been known for centuries; Hippocrates and Galen outlined its symptoms. Rembrandt, in his famous painting *Old Man*, skilfully described the appearance of a person with advanced atherosclerosis: hard, twisty blood vessels visible under the skin, a yellowish lipid ring around the iris of the eye, signs of poor circulation on the nose and cheeks, yellowish, fatty deposits around the eyes (called xanthelasma), hair loss and dry skin.[4,6]

Autopsy studies have found that, by the age of 60, 100% of people have some signs of atherosclerosis.[6] The older we become the more atherosclerotic features we accumulate. So, the question is whether atherosclerosis is a disease, or simply a normal part of the ageing process? Perhaps it is a normal part of ageing, but the problem is that more and more of our younger generations are falling prey to this disease, which is a sign of something going wrong, something that Nature did not intend.

Conventional medicine does not know what causes atherosclerosis or how to cure it. Risk factors have been identified that are thought to contribute to the development of atherosclerosis. However, they are only risk factors; they are not causes of the disease. Among them are smoking, obesity, diabetes, high blood pressure, physical inactivity, male gender, family history of arterial disease, stress and an anxious and aggressive personality. There are about 200 risk factors – and the list is still growing.[5,6,7]

However, the risk factors that people hear the most about are cholesterol and dietary fats. The popular media, doctors, pharmacists, government bodies and the food industry all keep telling us that cholesterol and dietary fats "cause" heart disease and all other manifestations of atherosclerosis. They tell us not to eat natural fats and natural foods containing cholesterol but to replace them with vegetable oils and margarine. They tell us to remove meats and eggs from the diet and replace them with carbohydrates. They initiated and keep promoting a fat paranoia in the population. They use powerful drugs and other procedures to reduce our blood cholesterol. They have been waging a war on cholesterol and fats for the last 40–50 years. Yet, the rates of atherosclerosis and heart disease are still steadily growing.[2,3,7] People all over the world are having just as many heart attacks and strokes as before, despite following "heart healthy" diets, exercising and taking "cholesterol pills". Marginally fewer of us are dying from heart attacks and strokes today because medicine has better ways of saving our lives when it comes to it. But heart disease and other manifestations of atherosclerosis show no signs of declining.[1,2,3,7] All the efforts of our medicine, our governments, our pharmaceutical industry and our food industry are not making any difference whatsoever. The "War on Heart Disease" that they declared decades ago is being lost. So, are we doing something wrong?

In this book we are going to try and understand what exactly atherosclerosis is and what *really* causes it. We will then look at what each and every one of us can do to prevent, and even reverse, atherosclerosis in our bodies. But before we get to those points we have to dispel some myths; myths that have become so ingrained in our society that people do not even question them any more. "Put your heart in your mouth" is an old expression meaning to be anxious or scared about something; so anxious that it feels as if your heart pounds in your throat and mouth. This expression gives a good indication of the whole attitude to heart disease in our modern world. In 1700 Sir Robert Walpole said, "When people will not weed their own minds, they are apt to be overrun with nettles." So, let us pull the nettles out to clear the way, so that we can see without obstructions what the reality is behind our heart disease epidemic.

Part One: THE MYTHS
The diet-heart hypothesis

The diet-heart hypothesis is the greatest scientific deception
of this century, perhaps of any century.

George Mann, eminent American physician and scientist

Everybody has heard about cholesterol and dietary fats "clogging up your arteries" and "causing heart disease". Even children have been told that cholesterol and fats are "bad". For decades we have been "educated" in that direction by the popular media, advertisements and labels on our food, such as "low fat", "no-fat", "low cholesterol", "no-cholesterol", "lowers your cholesterol", "protects your heart". Doctors are also convinced: cholesterol-lowering medications have become the most prescribed drugs in the world after painkillers. The pharmaceutical powers are now working very hard on an ultimate goal: to put everybody, including our children, on "preventative" cholesterol-lowering medication.

How did humanity manage to get to this situation? It is thanks to the **diet-heart hypothesis**, first proposed in 1953 by Ancel Keys, director of the Laboratory of Physiological Hygiene at the University of Minnesota. The hypothesis stated that dietary fats, including cholesterol, cause heart disease, and by avoiding these foods we can avoid developing heart disease.[1] In order to support this idea Ancel Keys made a diagram that showed the correlation of fat consumption and mortality from heart disease in six countries, which he carefully selected out of the 22 countries for which the data was available. This diagram showed a perfect correlation: the more fat consumed, the more deaths from heart disease. However, when all the remaining countries are added back to the diagram this correlation disappears. In fact the diagram now shows that there is no correlation between fat consumption and dying from heart disease.

Using Ancel Keys' method one can prove anything one likes. For example, let's say we want to prove that acne is caused by ... owning a hairdryer. To do that we collect data from as many countries as possible on how many people own a hairdryer and how many people suffer from acne. We plot all that data on a diagram, where the horizontal line shows the hairdryers and the vertical line shows the numbers of acne victims. We will finish up with a lot of dots, each representing a particular country. Then we pick those dots, that perfectly fit a line going up from left to right and we erase the rest of the dots. And, bingo, we have a diagram "proving" that acne is caused by owning a hairdryer! This is how Ancel Keys made his diagram. It is completely baffling as to why on earth the scientific community at the time accepted this kind of "scientific evidence." For whatever reason it did! That is how the diet-heart hypothesis started its long life – from a deception.

Russians have a proverb: "If there is no fish around, a shrimp will do". The heart disease epidemic was becoming an important public issue in the United States at that time, and the authorities were desperate to offer some explanation to the public to show that they were in control. So, when Ancel Keys proposed his hypothesis, it immediately appealed to politicians and the medical establishment, and money started pouring in. Institutions and laboratories were set up around the diet-heart hypothesis, thousands of people were employed and scientific grants were awarded to "prove" the hypothesis. The popular media followed by trumpeting the new "breakthrough". Once politicians and the public had bought the idea, the researchers had to come up with science to fit the bill. And so they set to work. No other medical hypothesis has been researched so much! Hundreds of studies have been conducted around the world to prove that dietary fat and cholesterol are the causes of heart disease. The Chinese have an old saying: "Cut the feet to fit the shoes". This is exactly what was done with a lot of studies in order to support the diet-heart hypothesis. The proponents used their data selectively: they ignored the data that did not support the hypothesis and inflated and advertised the data that did. In the meantime, for every study, that attempted to support the idea, honest studies were coming in from different countries proving it to be wrong. However, the political and commercial machine was in motion, and it was not prepared to stop.

As all this was going on, many renowned medics and honest scientists, who had the training to analyse the accumulated scientific data for themselves, opposed and criticised the diet-heart hypothesis and the "science" conducted to support it.

Dr Reiser, a former professor of biochemistry at Texas University, conducted a thorough review of almost all the experiments on the influence of dietary fatty acids on blood cholesterol. His conclusion was that most experiments were "biased by serious faults". He wrote: "One must be bold indeed to attempt to persuade large segments of the populations of the world to change their accustomed diets... with the results of such uncontrolled, primitive, trial-and-error type explorations."[2]

The late professor George Mann, former professor of medicine and biochemistry at Vanderbilt University in Tennessee, called the diet-heart hypothesis "the greatest scientific deception of our times". Talking about scientists who promote the diet-heart hypothesis he wrote: "Fearing to lose their soft money funding, the academicians who should speak up and stop this wasteful anti-science are strangely quiet. Their silence has delayed a solution for coronary heart disease by a generation."[3,13]

Dr Paul J Rosch, President of the American Institute of Stress, Clinical Professor of Medicine and Psychiatry at New York Medical College, Vice President of the International Stress Management Association and Chairman of its US branch wrote: "A massive crusade has been conceived to 'lower your cholesterol count' by rigidly restricting dietary fat, coupled with aggressive drug treatment. Much of the impetus for this comes from speculation, rather than any solid scientific proof... The cholesterol cartel of drug companies, manufacturers of low-fat foods, blood-testing devices and others with huge vested financial interests have waged a highly successful promotional campaign. Their power is so great that they have infiltrated medical and governmental regulatory agencies that would normally protect us from such unsubstantiated dogma".[4,5]

The late Dr Mary Enig, an international expert in lipid biochemistry, President of the Maryland Nutritionists Association and a consulting editor to the *Journal of the American College of Nutrition* and many other scientific publications, wrote: "The idea that saturated fats cause heart disease is completely wrong, but the statement has been 'published' so many times over the last three or more decades that it is very difficult to convince people otherwise unless they are willing to take the time to read and learn what all the economic and political facts were that produced the anti-saturated-fat agenda".[6]

Dr William E Stehbens, professor at the Department of Pathology, Wellington School of Medicine and director of the Malaghan Institute of Medical Research in Wellington, New Zealand, has conducted thorough reviews of studies around the diet-heart hypothesis. He wrote: "The lipid hypothesis has enjoyed undeserved longevity and respectability. Readers should be aware of the unscientific nature of claims used to support it and see it as little more than a pernicious bum steer.... Continued, unquestioned use of unreliable data has led to premature conclusions and the sacrifice of truth. The degree of inaccuracy of vital statistics for CHD is of such uncertain magnitude that, when superimposed on other deficiencies already indicated, the concept of an epidemic rise and decline of CHD in many countries must be regarded as unproven, and governmental or health policies based on unreliable data become completely untenable...The perpetuation of the cholesterol myth and the alleged preventive measures are doing the dairy and meat industries of this and other countries much harm quite apart from their potential to endanger optimum nutrition levels and the health of the populace at large".[7]

Dr Ray Rosenman, cardiologist, retired director of Cardiovascular Research in the Health Sciences Program at SRI International in Menlo Park, California and Associate Chief of Medicine, Mt. Zion Hospital and Medical Center in San Francisco, has published widely on the subject of cardiovascular disease. Here is his conclusion on all the science relating to the diet-heart hypothesis: "These data lead to a conclusion that neither diet, serum lipids, nor their changes can explain wide national and regional difference in heart disease rates, nor the variable 20th century rises and declines of CHD mortality...The preventive effects of dietary and drug treatments have been exaggerated by a tendency in trial reports, reviews, and other papers to cite and inflate supportive results, while suppressing discordant data, and many such examples are cited".[12]

The late Dr Russell Smith, an American experimental psychologist, participated in publishing two thorough reviews of the existing scien-

tific data on the diet-heart hypothesis with more than 3,000 references. His conclusion was: "The current campaign to convince every
American to change his or her diet and, in many cases, to initiate drug
'therapy' for life is based on fabrications, erroneous interpretations
and/or gross exaggerations of findings and, very importantly, the
ignoring of massive amounts of unsupportive data... It does not seem
possible that objective scientists without vested interests could ever
interpret the literature as supportive... It is depressing to know that
billions of dollars and a highly sophisticated medical research system
are being wasted chasing windmills".[8]

Professor Lars Werko, retired professor of medicine at Sahlgren's
Hospital, Gothenburg, Sweden and Head of the Swedish Council on
Technology Assessment in Health Care, heavily criticised the large
epidemiological studies that support the diet-heart hypothesis. He
concluded: "No studies have proved anything, but instead of formu-
lating new hypotheses, diet-heart supporters call the current one the
most probable truth, and they have intervened in people's lives
because they will not wait for the final proof".[9]

Dr Edward Pinckney, a former co-editor of the *Journal of the
American Medical Association,* in his book *The Cholesterol Controversy*
summarised: "If you have come to believe that you can ward off death
from heart disease by altering the amount of cholesterol in your blood,
whether by diet or by drugs, you are following a regime that still has
no basis in fact. Rather, you as a consumer have been taken in by
certain commercial interests and health groups who are more interested in your money than your life".[11]

The most comprehensive professional review of all available science
on this subject has been conducted by Dr Uffe Ravnskov, MD, PhD, and
published in his revolutionary book *The Cholesterol Myths* in 2000. His
conclusion was: "Masses of valid scientific evidence should have
destroyed the diet-heart idea by now. Yet, like the ancient Greek Hydra,
a mythological monster that grew new heads whenever its old ones
were chopped off, the cholesterol Hydra continues its life as if nothing
had happened... Scientists, who support the diet-heart idea and who
are honest must be ignorant, either because they have failed to understand what they have read or else, by blindly following the authorities,
they have failed to check the accuracy of the studies written by those

authorities. But some scientists must surely have realised that the diet-heart idea is impossible and yet, for various reasons, have chosen to keep the idea alive".[12]

Many of you would ask the logical questions: "Why don't doctors know better? Why does my doctor tell me to avoid eating fat and cholesterol and want to put me on cholesterol-lowering medication?" Dr Paul J Rosch answers this question very well: "Practising physicians get most of their information from the drug companies. Compared to their peers a half century ago, most doctors don't have the time or skills to critically evaluate reports, very few know anything about research, nor did the generation that taught them".[5] So, doctors know and understand no more about the diet-heart hypothesis than any member of the general public because they derive their information from the same source as the general public – commercial companies, who are making billions on this idea.

To support his hypothesis Dr Ancel Keys invented the term, "Mediterranean Diet", claiming that it is the best diet for your heart. This is how he described the Mediterranean diet: "The heart of what we now consider the Mediterranean diet is mainly vegetarian... Pasta in many forms, leaves sprinkled with olive oil, all kinds of vegetables in season, and often cheese, all finished off with fruit and frequently washed down with wine".[12] Anybody who has travelled to the Mediterranean countries will tell you that their diet is nothing like the one described by Dr Keys. Whether you are in Spain, France, Italy, Croatia, Greece, Cyprus, North Africa or anywhere else around the Mediterranean Sea, you will be served plenty of meats, fish, cheese, eggs, butter and nothing low fat. If you tell them that they are vegetarians, they will probably die from laughter.

It is also a myth that people in Mediterranean countries do not suffer from heart disease: there are great variations within each country and between different countries, regardless of how much fat they consume.[69]

But what about all the science?

There are internationally accepted rules for conducting credible science.

Dr Uffe Ravnskov, MD, explains: "If a scientific hypothesis is sound, it must agree with **all** observations. A hypothesis is not like a sports event, where the team with the greatest number of points wins the game. Even one observation that does not support a hypothesis is enough to disprove it. The proponents of a scientific idea have the burden of proof on their shoulders. The opponent does not have to present an alternative idea; his task is only to find the weakness in the hypothesis. If there is only one proof against it, one proof that cannot be denied and that is based on reliable scientific observations, the hypothesis must be rejected. And the diet-heart idea is filled with features that have repeatedly been proven false".[12]

Even one observation should be enough to disprove a hypothesis! But we have hundreds of studies that have provided us with plenty of evidence to show that the diet-heart hypothesis is a big mistake! The proponents of the diet-heart idea have been sweeping this evidence under the carpet for years. Now let us have a look at it.

1. In Britain fat consumption has been stable since 1910, while the number of heart attacks has increased 10 times between 1930 and 1970. So, in Britain, having a heart disease has nothing to do with how much fat you eat.[2,5,8,12,29]

2. Since World War II the Japanese have been eating more and more animal fat, while fewer and fewer of them die from heart attacks. On top of that, mortality from most diseases decreased in Japan as they ate more animal fat.[8,17,18]

3. In Switzerland, after World War II intake of animal fat increased by 20%, yet the death rate from heart disease steadily decreased. So, one can say that in Switzerland eating more fat helps against heart disease.[12,16]

4. In the USA, between 1930 and 1960, mortality from heart disease increased 10 times, while the consumption of animal fat decreased. Just from this data, one can create a hypothesis that reducing animal fat in your food causes heart disease.[11,12,30]

5. In Yugoslavia, between 1955 and 1965, the number of heart attacks increased 10 times, while fat intake reduced by 25%. One can conclude that in Yugoslavia eating less fat causes heart disease.[12]

6. The worriers in the indigenous Samburu and Masai tribes in Kenya largely subsist on meat, fat, milk and blood, they eat very little plant matter. Professor George Mann, from Vanderbilt University in Nashville, and other researchers have studied these people for many years. They found them to be free from any modern disease, including heart disease. Their blood cholesterol was very low, despite the fact that they gorged on fat and cholesterol daily. However, when these same people moved to the city of Nairobi and adopted a modern lifestyle with a modern low-fat diet, they became prone to heart disease, just like anybody else. The example of these people alone is enough to show that the diet-heart hypothesis is wrong.[3,11,13,14]

7. In India, studies by Dr S L Malhotra of Bombay have demonstrated that people in Madras, who eat very little fat and no animal fat at all, die from heart disease seven times more, and at a younger age, than people from Punjab, where traditionally a lot of animal fat is consumed. So again, animal fat appears to be heart protective.[11,12,23,30]

8. Dozens of studies have been conducted in different countries to discover whether people with heart disease eat more fat and cholesterol. Every study shows that they eat the same amount of fat and cholesterol as people without any heart disease.[7,9,10,12,15,19] By 1998 there had been 30 studies that clearly demonstrated that consuming animal fat has nothing to do with heart disease. However, these studies found that eating vegetable oils and margarine is strongly associated with heart disease.

9. Study after study has shown that people with a normal level of cholesterol die from heart disease just as often as people with high cholesterol, and that blood cholesterol level cannot predict a heart attack.[10,12,15,16,17,21,61]

10. Many studies clearly demonstrated that **low** cholesterol levels are associated with greater mortality from heart disease and other diseases.[10,15,18,23,24,27,30,61] So, people with low cholesterol are more likely to die early.

11. From the very beginnings of the diet-heart hypothesis, study after study has demonstrated that high cholesterol is not a risk factor for women.[10,11,12,15,24,31] In fact it has been shown that **low** choles-

terol is dangerous for women. Researchers in France found that old women with a high level of cholesterol live the longest and healthiest lives, while women with low cholesterol are five times more likely to die early.[11,12,27,28,30,62] The French researchers warned against cholesterol lowering in women, particularly in old age, when cholesterol has been shown to be health protective. So, women should stop worrying about their cholesterol level at all. And yet doctors don't seem to be aware of this fact because they prescribe cholesterol-lowering medication to women just as much as they do to men, and typically it is the older women who get the prescription. Incidentally, what women need to worry about is cancer, as it kills almost twice as many women under the age of 75 than heart disease does.[12]

12. High cholesterol in men had no association with heart disease in many studies.[10,12,15,16,17,18,21,57,61] In fact, the majority of studies show that men, just like women, die more from heart disease and other health problems if they have low cholesterol levels. And yet doctors are busy prescribing cholesterol-lowering medication to millions of men around the world.

13. In Russia, low cholesterol has been shown to be associated with an increased risk of heart disease.[12,30,61] Again, cholesterol appears to be heart protective.

14. Many studies have shown that, in old age, cholesterol is protective: old people with high cholesterol live longer than people with low cholesterol. In fact, it is dangerous to reduce cholesterol in old people.[12,27,59,60,62]

15. Study after study in many countries has demonstrated that it is impossible to reduce your blood cholesterol or the death rate from heart disease by a low-fat, low-cholesterol diet. In fact, animal fat and cholesterol in the food we eat have virtually no effect on the level of our blood cholesterol.[10,11,15,16,17,18,25] Why? Because every organ and every cell of the body can produce cholesterol. When we eat lots of cholesterol, the body produces less; when we eat less cholesterol, the body produces more. Of course, the food industry would not like you to know this fact.

16. At least 60% of the people who have heart attacks have normal levels of blood cholesterol.[11,12,29,30]

17. Children on low-fat diets suffer from growth problems, failure to thrive and learning disabilities. Incidentally, in children no connection was found between what they eat and their blood cholesterol levels.[12,22,30,37,38,58,63]

18. People in France, Germany, Austria and Luxembourg have high levels of cholesterol, and yet the death rates from heart disease are very low in these countries.[12,64]

19. The supporters of the diet-heart hypothesis often point to Japan, claiming that their low-fat diet results in low mortality from heart disease. In Japan, it is traditionally considered shameful to die from heart disease, so Japanese doctors rarely put a diagnosis of heart disease on a death certificate.[12] That is why heart disease mortality in Japan is usually recorded as low. Japanese who immigrate to Western countries generally have the same mortality from heart disease as the Western population. Incidentally, Japanese immigrants who maintain their low-fat diet die from heart attacks twice as often as those who adopt a Western high-fat diet.[12,17,18]

20. Large clinical trials where patients were put on a low-fat, low-cholesterol, high-carbohydrate, vegetarian diet created a drastically increased risk of heart disease.[16,18,20,23,24] The author of one study at Harvard Medical School, Dr L Gould, one of the United States' leading cardiologists, concluded: "I do not recommend a high-carbohydrate strict vegetarian diet as it incurs substantial risk of coronary events".[21]

21. Study after study has clearly demonstrated that there is no correlation between the level of blood cholesterol and the degree of atherosclerosis: people with low cholesterol can be just as sclerotic as people with high cholesterol.[10,12,15,26,27]

22. The gigantic-scale American MRFIT study found that people who ate less animal fat and cholesterol had higher blood cholesterol.[10] This finding has been quietly forgotten by the proponents of the diet-heart hypothesis. The explanation for their finding is the fact that when we eat less cholesterol the body produces more, because our human bodies cannot live without cholesterol. The director of another huge project – the Framingham Heart Study – has concluded, "In Framingham the more saturated fat one ate, the more cholesterol one ate, the more calories one ate, the lower the

person's serum cholesterol... We found that the people who ate the most cholesterol, ate the most saturated fat, ate the most calories, weighed the least and were the most physically active".[15] So, eating animal fats and cholesterol was shown to be essential to being fit, trim and active.

23. Starting from the Framingham study, many large-scale studies have found that people who had **low** levels of cholesterol were prone to cancer.[15] A great number of studies found that cholesterol tends to be low for many years in a person before cancer is diagnosed.[10,12,15,30,66,67] So, having low cholesterol is dangerous, and in further chapters of this book we will see why. Yet, the public is led to believe that cholesterol is such an evil that the lower it is the better.

24. The MRFIT study,[10] the Lipid Research Clinics Programme[65] and many other studies have shown that you cannot reduce blood cholesterol by diet. The only way to reduce blood cholesterol is by using drugs.[10,12,15,19,23,24,28,38,54]

25. Most studies where blood cholesterol was reduced by using cholesterol-lowering drugs, such as gemfibrozil, colestipol and cholestyramine, showed that, despite the low cholesterol, people on these drugs died from heart disease just as often as those without any medication.[12,23,28,29,32] However, in those who took the drug, a drastic increase in cases of violent death and suicide has been reported. On top of that, these drugs cause very unpleasant side effects: abdominal pain, nausea, vomiting, heartburn, stomach ulcers, constipation and diarrhoea.

26. Another frightening chapter in the diet-heart saga is an operation, where a large part of the person's intestine, the ileum, is surgically removed. That is the part of our digestive system, which absorbs bile and cholesterol in order for the body to reuse these vital substances. When you remove the ileum the level of blood cholesterol goes down dramatically. A surgeon at the University of Minnesota, Dr H Bushwald, came up with this bright idea in 1963, and consequently conducted hundreds of this kind of operation. Some surgeons in other countries followed suit. The result of this activity was a lot of digestive side effects, repeated operations to correct them, malabsorption, increased incidence of kidney stones,

gall bladder problems, bowel obstructions and .... about the same mortality from heart disease in both operated and control groups. The operations reduced cholesterol but operated people died from heart disease just as much as people who had no operation.[5,12,16,68] So, this mutilating operation did not provide any protection from heart disease after all.

27. New cholesterol-lowering drugs, called statins, were introduced in the late 1980s. Some of the most commonly used ones are simvastatin, atorvastatin, fluvastatin and pravastatin. These drugs inhibit the body's ability to produce cholesterol and as a result effectively lower the blood cholesterol level. As a result, the list of side effects they cause is long. Statins produce an increased risk of cancer development, breast cancer in particular, in animals and humans.[4,5,11,32,38,81] Other side effects include liver damage, nerve damage, short temper, cognitive decline, memory loss and violent behaviour.[37,38,47,48,79,81] Taking statins during pregnancy may lead to more serious malformations in the baby than were seen after exposure to thalidomide.[35,37,38,79] These drugs can cause kidney failure, which has already claimed the lives of several hundred people, and resulted in one of the statins, cerivastatin, being withdrawn from the market. [2,38] Muscle damage can be a very serious side effect, particularly when the heart muscle is affected, as this can lead to heart failure.[33,35,38, 39] Statins block the synthesis of the coenzyme Q10, an essential chemical for energy production in the body. Statins are the number one profit-makers for the pharmaceutical industry; they have already become the most prescribed drugs in the Western world after painkillers. As Dr Malcolm Kendrick, MD (UK), has put it: "We are sleep-walking into what could become a major medical disaster because statin drugs will soon be sold over-the-counter".[38] Memory loss is a very serious result of statin therapy.[36, 37, 38,79,81] In fact, it is possible that a considerable part of the memory-loss (dementia) epidemic in our ageing population is due to our ubiquitous statin prescriptions. Our human brain is very cholesterol hungry; it takes some 25% of all body cholesterol and uses it for many vital jobs. Statins rob the brain of cholesterol, and hence the brain cannot function properly.[70,79] Statins have been linked to the development of

Parkinson's disease. Dr Xuemei Huang, from North Carolina University, having researched the connection, commented: "A surge in Parkinson's disease could be imminent because of the widespread use of statins".[80]

28. Cholesterol protects us from infections. People with low blood cholesterol are more prone to infections,[72,73,76] and when they get an infection they have an increased risk of dying from it compared to people with high cholesterol.[71,74,75] When people with low cholesterol and suppressed immunity were fed high-cholesterol foods their ability to fight infection was substantially boosted.[75] For centuries before the discovery of antibiotics, a mixture of raw egg yolks and cream, very rich in cholesterol, was used as a cure for tuberculosis. Cholesterol supports immunity in laboratory studies by inactivating microbial toxins and assisting various parts of the immune system in fighting the infection.[77,78]

29. From the beginning of cholesterol-lowering trials, an increased number of deaths from violence and suicide have been recorded. Historically, from animal and human studies it is known that low blood cholesterol is associated with aggressive behaviour and suicide.[34,47,53,54] Low blood cholesterol has been routinely recorded in criminals who committed murder and other violent crimes, people with aggressive and violent personalities, people prone to suicide and people with aggressive social behaviour and low self-control.[12,47,48,53] The late Oxford professor, David Horrobin, in one of his publications warned us: "reducing cholesterol in the population on a large scale could lead to a general shift to more violent patterns of behaviour. Most of this increased violence would not result in death but in more aggression at work and in the family, more child abuse, more wife-beating and generally more unhappiness".[12,47]

30. The MRFIT study, Japanese and other studies have shown that low blood cholesterol is associated with a high risk of brain haemorrhage or stroke.[10,12,17,20,23,57] The older the person, the more their low blood cholesterol poses a risk of stroke, while it has been clearly demonstrated that high blood cholesterol protects older people from strokes, heart disease, infections and many other health problems.[12,27,59,60,62] Uffe Ravnskov poses a question:

"Perhaps we should take steps to raise the blood cholesterol in older people rather than lower it?"[12] Instead, our medical system is busy putting nearly every old person on "cholesterol pills" to lower their cholesterol.

31. The proponents of the diet-heart hypothesis and public policy-makers tell us that our children, from the age of two, should follow a programme for reducing their blood cholesterol by avoiding natural fats and replacing them with margarine. The pharmaceutical giants are working hard to create cholesterol-lowering drugs for children. These dangerous guidelines are given out "just in case", without any scientific data to support them.[12,20,21,54,58,63] Having looked at all the dangers of low-fat diet and reducing blood cholesterol, it is easy to see that the consequences of this policy can be very serious indeed for our children: aggressive behaviour, learning difficulties, poor memory, poor immunity, poor physical health combined with the future risk of developing cancer, heart disease, stroke and infertility.

32. As the proponents of the diet-heart hypothesis had told the world not to eat animal fats, they had to replace them with something. So, they proposed vegetable oils, such as corn oil, soy oil, canola oil, peanut oil, rapeseed oil and sunflower oil, and the solid fats made from these oils: margarines and shortenings. When Mother Nature made us, humans, she provided us with all the foods right for our physiology. But we have to eat them in the form Nature produced them. Seeds, nuts and other plant matter contain polyunsaturated fatty acids, which are very fragile; they are easily damaged by heat, light, exposure to oxygen and other factors. When we chew seeds in their natural form we get oils from them in their natural state, unadulterated and in small amounts. When these oils are expressed from plants on a commercial scale, solvents and very high temperatures are used, which damage the chemical structure of the oils. Never in human history has our physiology been exposed to such amounts of chemically altered vegetable oils as in these last few decades, thanks to the diet-heart hypothesis. Our bodies have not been designed to use these kinds of fat. We have accumulated plenty of solid scientific evidence to show that these chemically changed fats cause cancer, heart

disease, diabetes, neurological damage, immune abnormalities and other health problems.[40,43,44,45,46] To make vegetable oils into solid margarine, they have to be hydrogenated, which creates a new kind of fat that is even more dangerous for our health. These oils and margarines have been vigorously promoted by the food industry for decades now as a "healthy" replacement for natural butter and animal fats. And yet, from the beginning of this promotion campaign, study after study has shown that these oils and margarines are dangerous. First it was discovered that these oils damage our white blood cells, making us more prone to infections, inflammation and cancer.[43,44,46] Vegetable oils and margarine accelerate ageing.[42,43] Animals fed these oils develop brain damage, testicular abnormalities and infertility.[40,45] Premature children fed a formula rich in these fats develop anaemia, oedema, damage to blood cells and lack of vitamin E.[40,41,43]

One particular group of these chemically changed fats, called trans fats, is now receiving quite a lot of attention.[42,43,46,49,50,51,52] They inhibit the functioning of normal fatty acids in the body, interfering in a myriad of normal processes in our cells. Trans fats have been found to have a damaging effect on our cardiovascular system, immune system, reproductive system, energy metabolism, fat and essential fatty acid metabolism, liver function and cell membranes.[46,49,50,52] They can cause heart disease, cancer, auto-immunity, infertility in men and women and interfere with pregnancy.[82] A pregnant woman who consumes trans fats passes them to her foetus. It has been found that these babies are more likely to be born premature with low birth weight and a high concentration of trans fatty acids in their blood.[49,82] It is possible that the wide consumption of vegetable oils is partly responsible for the growing number of our babies born prematurely.

The proponents of the diet-heart hypothesis have promoted vegetable oils in order to reduce cholesterol. The surprise for them was that study after study found that, instead of reducing blood cholesterol, these oils increase it.[46,47,50,52] They also cause athero-sclerosis in experiments.[53,55,56] Despite all this data vegetable oils and margarine are still being advertised as "healthy and heart protective". All the processed foods cooked with these oils and margarines such as baked and fried goods, crisps, snacks, biscuits, cakes, ready meals, sauces and condiments, will provide you with plenty of these chemically mutilated fats. It has been estimated that an average adult in the West now consumes 20–60g of trans fats a day.[12,46,51,52,82] Is it a surprise then that the Western population suffers from epidemics of all the diseases associated with these fats?

However, there are some plant oils that are good for us. *Cold-pressed* olive oil, made according to time-proven traditional methods, is one of those oils. It is full of health-giving properties, as long as it has not been heated at any stage. Cooking with olive oil is not a good idea because the heat destroys a lot of vitamins, antioxidants and other nutritious substances and changes some unsaturated fatty acids into harmful trans fats. Apart from olive oil, we have many other cold-pressed vegetable oils on the market: flax seed oil, avocado oil, hemp seed oil, evening primrose oil and walnut oil, as well as mixtures of different oils. All these oils contain very fragile unsaturated fatty acids, which need to be treated with great care in order not to turn them into harmful trans fats and other chemically altered fats.[82] They need to be cold expressed under very strict conditions, refrigerated at all times and kept away from light, heat and oxygen. Obviously, they must never be used for cooking. Providing that all these conditions are met, these oils have been shown to be beneficial for health when used as nutritional supplements in small amounts. Unfortunately, these good oils are not consumed by the majority of the population in the West. The majority gorges on dangerous margarines, vegetable oils and cooking oils without any idea of what they are doing to their health.

Looking at all the evidence, any thinking person would ask: "How on earth could international science accept the diet-heart hypothesis? And not only accept, but carry on promoting it for decades?"

To answer these questions I would quote Dr Uffe Ravnskov, MD, "One of my objections to the diet-heart idea is that its proponents are selective about their data. They lean on studies that support their idea – or that they claim, not always truthfully, support it – and ignore those that contradict them... Unfortunately, this happens all too frequently. Researchers get a result that is contrary to the cholesterol hypothesis, and yet they write conclusions indicating that their findings are in support. These misleading conclusions are most often written up in the summary of the papers, the only part of the paper that most doctors and researchers are likely to read. To find the contradictory results, you have to read the whole paper and meticulously study the tables".[12]

This is the story of the diet-heart hypothesis: it began its life from a deception and so it continues. Because doctors and policy-makers have no time or training to examine the papers themselves, they rely on summaries of the papers, which turn out to be deceptive. The medical, political and scientific establishments have long married themselves to the diet-heart hypothesis. To admit that they were wrong would do too much damage to their reputation, so they are not going to do it. In the meantime, their closed ranks give complete freedom to commercial companies to exploit the diet heart hypothesis to their advantage. Their relentless propaganda through the popular media ensures long life for this thoroughly discredited idea, which is doing immeasurable damage to the health of people all over the world.

But let us be optimistic! Human history is littered with stories of various mistaken theories and hypotheses, proposed by the most learned men of the time. On average it takes humanity 50 to 60 years to find the mistake and correct it. I have no doubt that, in the next couple of decades, the diet-heart hypothesis will be dismissed and laughed at as one of those mistakes!

Cholesterol: friend or foe?

The art of medicine consists in amusing the patient while nature cures the disease.

Voltaire

In our modern world, cholesterol has become almost a swear word. Thanks to the promoters of the diet-heart hypothesis, everybody "knows" that cholesterol is "evil" and has to be fought at every turn. If you believe the popular media you would think that there is simply no level of cholesterol low enough. If you are over a certain age you are likely to be tested for how much cholesterol you have in your blood. If it is higher than about 7–8 mmol/l (270mg/100ml), you may be prescribed a "cholesterol pill". Millions of people around the world take these pills, thinking that this way they are taking good care of their health. What these people don't know is just how far from the truth they are.

The truth is that we humans cannot live without cholesterol. Let us see why?

Our bodies are made out of billions of cells. Almost every cell produces cholesterol all the time during all of our lives. Why? Because every cell of every organ has cholesterol as part of its structure.[1,2,3] Cholesterol is an integral and very important part of our cell membranes; the membranes that make the cell wall and the walls of all organelles inside the cell. What is cholesterol doing there? A number of things.

First of all saturated fats and cholesterol make the walls of the cells firm – without them the cells will become flabby and fluid.[4] If we humans didn't have cholesterol and saturated fats in the walls of our cells, we would look like giant worms or slugs. And we are not talking about a few molecules of cholesterol here and there. In many cells, almost half of the cell wall is made from cholesterol.[2,5] Different kinds of cells in the body need different amounts of cholesterol, depending on their function and purpose. If the cell is part of a protective barrier, it will have a lot of cholesterol in it to make it strong, sturdy and resistant to any invasion. If a cell or an organelle inside the cell needs to be soft and fluid, it will have less cholesterol in its walls.[2,4]

This ability of cholesterol and saturated fats to firm and reinforce the tissues in the body is used by our blood vessels, particularly those that have to withstand the high pressure and turbulence of the blood flow. These are usually large or medium arteries in places where they divide or bend.[6,7] The flow of blood pounding through these arteries forces them to incorporate a layer of cholesterol and saturated fat in the wall, which makes it stronger, tougher and more rigid. These layers of cholesterol and fat are called *fatty streaks*. They are completely normal and form in all of us, starting from birth and sometimes even before we are born.[8] Various indigenous populations around the world, who never suffer from heart disease, have been found to have plenty of fatty streaks in their blood vessels in young and old, including children.[7] Fatty streaks do not belong to a disease, called atherosclerosis, which we will discuss in the next chapter.[6,7,8]

All the cells in our bodies have to communicate with each other. How do they do that? They use proteins embedded into the wall of the cell.[1,3] How are these proteins fixed to the wall? With the help of cholesterol and saturated fats! Cholesterol and stiff saturated fatty acids form so-called *lipid rafts*, which make little homes for every protein in the membrane and allow it to perform its functions.[1,2,4,9] Without cholesterol and saturated fats our cells would not be able to communicate with each other or transport various molecules into and out of the cell. As a result, our bodies would not be able to function the way they do.

The human brain is particularly rich in cholesterol: 8–22% of dry weight of different parts of the human brain is cholesterol [64] and around 25% of all body cholesterol is taken by the brain.[10,11,14] Every cell and every structure in the brain and the rest of our nervous system needs cholesterol, not only to build itself but also to accomplish its many functions. The developing brain and eyes of the foetus and a newborn infant require large amounts of cholesterol.[13,14] If the foetus doesn't get enough cholesterol during development the child may be born with a congenital abnormality called a cyclopean eye.[12] Human breast milk provides a lot of cholesterol (around 31mg/100ml in the colostrum and 3–19mg/100ml in the milk).[4,34,35] Not only that, mother's milk provides a specific enzyme to allow the baby's digestive tract to absorb almost 100% of that cholesterol, because the developing brain and eyes of an infant require large amounts of it.[4,12,13,34,35] Children deprived of cholesterol in infancy may end up with poor eyesight and brain function.[14] Manufacturers of infant formulas are aware of this fact, but following the anti-cholesterol dogma, they produce formulas with virtually no cholesterol in them.

One of the most abundant materials in the brain and the rest of our nervous system is a fatty substance called myelin.[3,4,5] Myelin coats every nerve cell and every nerve fibre like an insulating cover around electric wires. Apart from insulation, it provides nourishment and protection for every tiny structure in our brain and the rest of the nervous system. People who start losing their myelin develop a condition called multiple sclerosis. Well, around 20% of the dry weight of myelin is cholesterol.[4,11,64] If you start interfering with the body's ability to produce cholesterol, you put the very structure of the brain and the rest of the nervous system under threat. The synthesis of myelin in the brain is tightly connected with the synthesis of cholesterol.[10,11] In my clinical experience, foods with high cholesterol and high animal fat content are an essential medicine for a person with multiple sclerosis or any other nervous system disorder.

One of the most wonderful abilities we humans are blessed with is an ability to remember things – our human memory. How do we form memories? By our brain cells establishing connections with each other, called synapses.[3] The more healthy synapses a person's brain can make, the more mentally able and intelligent that person is. Scientists have discovered that synapse formation is almost entirely dependent on cholesterol, which is produced by the brain cells in a form of "apolipoprotein E".[11,15] Without the presence of this factor we cannot form synapses, and hence we would not be able to learn or remember anything. Memory loss is one of the side effects of cholesterol-lowering drugs.[6,16] In my clinic I see growing numbers of people with memory loss who have been taking "cholesterol pills". Dr Duane Graveline, MD, former NASA scientist and astronaut, suffered such memory loss while taking his "cholesterol pill". He managed to save his memory by stopping the pill and eating lots of cholesterol-rich foods. Since then he has described his experience in his book *Lipitor –*

Thief of Memory, Statin Drugs and the Misguided War on Cholesterol.[16] Dietary cholesterol in fresh eggs and other cholesterol-rich foods has been shown in scientific trials to improve memory in the elderly.[4,6] In my clinical experience, any person with memory loss or learning problems needs to have plenty of these foods every single day in order to recover.

Let us see which foods are rich in cholesterol.[3,4,5,17,18]

1. Just like our own human brain, brains of animals are rich in cholesterol. Animal brains are the richest food source of cholesterol, providing from 3100mg cholesterol (per 100g of beef brain) to 1352mg of cholesterol (per 100g of lamb brain).[4,5,17] In traditional cultures brain of animals was considered to be a delicacy and was known to be very beneficial for health.

2. Organ meats are rich in cholesterol. Veal kidney can provide 791mg per 100g while chicken liver can provide 563mg per 100g. Other organ meats – liver and kidneys of other animals, heart, tongue, tripe, pancreas, foie gras and giblets will all provide good amounts of cholesterol.[4,5,17] Organ meats have always been considered to be health foods and sacred foods in traditional cultures all over the world.

3. Caviar (fish eggs) is the next richest source; it provides 588mg of cholesterol per 100g.[5,18]

4. Cod liver oil follows closely with 570mg of cholesterol per 100g. There is no doubt that the cholesterol element of cod liver oil plays an important role in all the well-known health benefits of this time-honoured health food.[17]

5. Fresh egg yolk takes the next place, with 424mg of cholesterol per 100g. I would like to repeat – fresh egg yolk, not chemically mutilated egg powders (they contain chemically mutilated cholesterol)![4,17]

6. Butter provides a good 218mg of cholesterol per 100g. We are talking about natural butter, not butter substitutes.[4,17]

7. Cold-water fish and shellfish, such as salmon, sardines, herring, mackerel and shrimps, provide good amounts of cholesterol, ranging from 173mg to 81mg per 100g. The proponents of low-cholesterol diets tell you to replace meats with fish. Obviously, they are

not aware of the fact that fish can be almost twice as rich in cholesterol than meats.[17,18]

8. Lard provides 94mg of cholesterol per 100g. Other animal fats
   follow.[4,18]

These foods give the body a hand in supplying cholesterol so it does
not have to work as hard to produce its own. What many people don't
realise is that most cholesterol in the body does not come from food!
The body produces cholesterol as it is needed.[3,5] Scientific studies have
conclusively demonstrated that cholesterol from food has virtually no
effect on the level of our blood cholesterol.[6] Why? Because cholesterol
is such an essential part of our human physiology that the body has
very efficient mechanisms to keep blood cholesterol at a certain level.
When we eat more cholesterol, the body produces less; when we eat
less cholesterol, the body produces more.[2,4,6] As a raw material for
making cholesterol the body can use carbohydrates, proteins and fats,
which means that your pasta and bread can be used for making cholesterol in the body.[5] It has been estimated that, in an average person,
about 85% of blood cholesterol is produced by the body, while only
15% comes from food.[6,27] So, even if you religiously follow a
completely cholesterol-free diet, you will still have a lot of cholesterol
in your body. However, cholesterol-lowering drugs are a completely
different matter! They interfere with the body's ability to produce
cholesterol, and hence they do reduce the amount of cholesterol available for the body to use.[6,16,19]

If we do not take cholesterol-lowering drugs, most of us don't have
to worry about cholesterol.[31,32] However, there are people whose
bodies, for various reasons, are unable to produce enough cholesterol.[6,20,22,30,33] These people are prone to emotional instability and
behavioural problems.[21,22] Low blood cholesterol has been routinely
recorded in criminals who have committed murder and other violent
crimes, people with aggressive and violent personalities, people prone
to suicide and people with aggressive social behaviour and low self-
control.[21,22,23] In this chapter I would like to repeat what the late
Oxford professor David Horrobin warned us about: "reducing cholesterol in the population on a large scale could lead to a general shift to
more violent patterns of behaviour. Most of this increased violence

would not result in death but in more aggression at work and in the family, more child abuse, more wife-beating and generally more unhappiness".[20] People whose bodies are unable to produce enough cholesterol do need to have plenty of foods rich in cholesterol in order to provide their organs with this essential-to-life substance.

What else does our body need all that cholesterol for?

After the brain the organs, most hungry for cholesterol, are our endocrine glands: adrenals and sex glands.[3,4,5,10] They produce steroid hormones. Steroid hormones in the body are made from cholesterol: testosterone, progesterone, pregnenolone, androsterone, oestrone, estradiol, corticosterone, aldosterone and others.[4,6,10] These hormones accomplish a myriad of functions in the body, from regulation of our metabolism, energy production, mineral assimilation, brain, muscle and bone formation to behaviour, emotions and reproduction. Our stressful modern lives consume a lot of these hormones, leading to a condition called "adrenal exhaustion". This condition is diagnosed a lot by naturopaths and other health practitioners. There are many herbal preparations on the market for adrenal exhaustion. However, the most important therapeutic measure is to provide your adrenal glands with plenty of dietary cholesterol.

Without cholesterol we would not be able to have children because every sex hormone in our bodies is made from cholesterol.[24,25,26,30] A fair percentage of our infertility epidemic can be laid at the doorstep of the "diet-heart hypothesis". The more eager we became to fight animal fats and cholesterol, the more problems with normal sexual development, fertility and reproduction we started to face.[26,27] A large percentage of Western men and women are infertile, and increasing numbers of our youngsters are growing up with abnormalities in their sex hormones. These abnormalities lead to many physical problems, abnormal sexual behaviour and sex crimes. Recent research has "discovered" that eating full-cream dairy products cures infertility in women.[26] Researchers found that women who drink whole milk and eat high-fat dairy products are more fertile than those who stick to low-fat products. Dr Jorge Chavarro, of the Harvard School of Public Health, who led the study published in *Human Reproduction*, emphasised: "Women wanting to conceive should examine their diet. They should consider changing low-fat dairy foods for high-fat dairy foods, for instance by swapping skimmed milk for whole milk and eating cream, not low-fat yoghurt".[26]

One of the busiest organs in terms of cholesterol production in our bodies is the liver. It regulates the level of our blood cholesterol.[3,4,10] Apart from that it puts a lot of cholesterol into bile production. Yes, cholesterol is one of the most important parts of bile.[3] Without bile we would not be able to digest and absorb fats and fat-soluble vitamins. Bile emulsifies fats, in other words, it mixes them with water, so that digestive enzymes can get to them. After it completes its mission most of the bile gets reabsorbed in the digestive system and brought back to the liver for recycling. In fact, 95% of our bile is recycled because the building blocks of bile, one of which is cholesterol, are too precious for the body to waste.[3,4,6] Nature doesn't do anything without good reason. This example alone of the careful recycling of cholesterol should have given us a good idea about its importance for the body!

Bile is essential for absorbing fat-soluble vitamins: vitamin A, vitamin D, vitamin K and vitamin E.[27,28] We cannot live without these vitamins. Apart from ensuring that fat-soluble vitamins get digested and absorbed properly, cholesterol is the major building block of one of these vitamins – vitamin D.[5,29] Vitamin D is made from cholesterol in our skin, when it is exposed to sunlight. In those times of the year when there isn't much sunlight we can get this vitamin from cholesterol-rich foods: organ meats, cod liver oil, fish, shellfish, butter, lard and eggs. Our recent misguided fear of sun and avoidance of cholesterol-rich foods have created an epidemic of vitamin D deficiency in the Western world.[39,40]

What does it mean for our bodies to be deficient in vitamin D?

A long list of suffering:[29,36,37,38]

- Diabetes, as vitamin D is essential for blood sugar control.
- Heart disease.
- Mental illness.
- Auto-immune illness, such as rheumatoid arthritis, lupus, inflammatory bowel disease, multiple sclerosis and others.
- Obesity.
- Osteoarthritis and osteoporosis.
- Rickets and osteomalacia.

- Muscle weakness and poor neuro-muscular co-ordination.
- High blood pressure.
- Cancer.
- Chronic pain.
- Poor immunity and susceptibility to infections.
- Hyperparathyroidism, which manifests itself as osteoporosis, kidney stones, depression, aches and pains, chronic fatigue, muscle weakness and digestive abnormalities.

Unfortunately, apart from sunlight and cholesterol-rich foods there is no other appropriate way to get vitamin D.[29,30,31,32,39,40] Of course, there are supplements, but most of them contain synthetic vitamin D. This vitamin is not the same as the natural vitamin D. It does not work as effectively and it is easy to get a toxic level of it.[29,39] In fact, almost all cases of vitamin D toxicity ever recorded were cases where synthetic vitamin D had been used. It is impossible to get toxicity from natural vitamin D obtained from sunlight or cholesterol-rich foods, because the body knows how to deal with an excess of those things. What the body does not know how to deal with is an excess of synthetic vitamin D.

Vitamin D has been designed to work as a team with another fat-soluble vitamin – vitamin A.[4,29,39] That is why foods rich in one are rich in the other. So, by eating organ meats, butter and eggs, for example, we can obtain both vitamins at the same time.

As we grow older, our ability to produce vitamin D in the skin under sunlight can be diminished.[29] So, taking foods rich in vitamin D is particularly important for older people. For the rest of us, sensible sunbathing is a wonderful, healthy and enjoyable way of getting a good supply of vitamin D. The skin cancer, blamed on sunshine, is not caused by the sun.[4,41,42,43,44,45,46,47,48] It is caused by trans fats from vegetable oils and margarine and other man-made toxins stored in the skin. In addition, many of the sunscreens that people use, contain chemicals, which have been proven to cause skin cancer.[42,43,44,48]

Cholesterol is essential for our immune system to function properly.[54,56] Animal experiments and human studies have demonstrated that immune cells rely on cholesterol in fighting infections and repairing themselves after the fight.[49] On top of that, LDL (low-density lipoprotein) cholesterol, or so-called "bad" cholesterol, directly binds and inactivates dangerous bacterial toxins, preventing them from doing any damage in the body. One of the most lethal toxins is produced by a widely spread bacterium, *Staphylococcus aureus*, which is the cause of MRSA, a common hospital infection. This toxin can literally dissolve red blood cells. However, it does not work in the presence of LDL cholesterol.[52] People who fall prey to this toxin have low blood cholesterol. Considering that today almost all older patients in our hospitals are prescribed statins to reduce their blood cholesterol, it is no wonder that MRSA has become such a problem as a hospital infection. In order to deal with it effectively we need to take steps **to increase** the cholesterol level in our hospital patients. It has been recorded that people with high levels of cholesterol are protected from infections: they are four times less likely to contract AIDS,[53,55] they rarely get common colds,[6,50] and they recover from infections more quickly than people with "normal" or low blood cholesterol.[51] On the other side of the spectrum, people with low blood cholesterol are prone to various infections, suffer from them longer and are more likely to die from an infection.[6,51] A diet rich in cholesterol has been demonstrated to improve these people's ability to recover from infections.[56] So, any person suffering from an acute or chronic infection needs to eat high-cholesterol foods to recover. Cod liver oil, rich in cholesterol, has long been prized as a remedy for the immune system. Those familiar with old medical literature will tell you that until the discovery of antibiotics a common cure for tuberculosis was a daily mixture of raw egg yolks and fresh cream.[57]

The questions are: Why do some people have more cholesterol in their blood than others? And why can the same person have different levels of cholesterol at different times of the day? Why is our level of cholesterol different in different seasons of the year: generally in winter it goes up and in the summer it goes down?[4] Why is it that blood cholesterol goes through the roof in people after any surgery?[31] Why does blood cholesterol go up when we have an infection?[51] Why does it go up after dental treatment?[32] Why does it go up when we are under stress?[31] And why does it become normal when we are relaxed and feel well?

The answer to all these questions is this: cholesterol is a healing agent in the body.[4,6,31,32,58] When the body has some healing jobs to do, it produces cholesterol and sends it to the site of the damage. Depending on the time of day, the weather, the season and our exposure to various environmental factors, the damage to various tissues in the body varies. As a result, the production of cholesterol in the body also varies.

Since we are talking about heart disease and atherosclerosis, let us look at blood vessels. Their inside walls are covered by a layer of cells called the endothelium.[3,10] Any damaging agent we are exposed to sooner or later finishes up in our bloodstream. Whether it is a toxic chemical, an infectious organism, a free radical or anything else, once it is in the blood what is it going to attack first? The endothelium, of course. The endothelium immediately sends a message to the liver. Whenever our liver receives a signal that a wound has been inflicted upon the endothelium somewhere in our vascular system, it gets into gear and sends cholesterol to the site of the damage in a shuttle, called LDL (low-density lipoprotein).[59] Because this cholesterol travels from the liver to the wound in the form of LDL, our "science", in its wisdom, called LDL a "bad" cholesterol. When the wound heals and the cholesterol is removed, it travels back to the liver in the form of HDL (high-density lipoprotein). Because this cholesterol travels away from the artery back to the liver, our misguided "science" called it "good" cholesterol.[6,59] This is like calling an ambulance travelling from the base to the patient, a "bad ambulance", and the one travelling from the patient back to the base, a "good ambulance". And that is not all. The latest thing that our science has "discovered" is that not all LDL cholesterol is so bad. Most of it is actually good. So, now we are told to call that part of LDL the "good bad cholesterol" and the rest of it the "bad bad cholesterol".[6,59,60]

Why does the liver send cholesterol to the site of the injury? Because the body cannot clear the infection, remove toxic elements or heal the wound without cholesterol and fats. Any healing involves the birth, growth and functioning of thousands of cells: immune cells, endothelial cells and many others. As these cells, to a considerable degree, are made out of cholesterol and fats, they cannot be born and grow without a good supply of these substances.[1,2,3,34] When the cells are damaged, they require cholesterol and fats to repair themselves. It is a scientific fact that any scar tissue in the body contains high amounts of cholesterol.[61] Another scientific fact is that cholesterol acts as an antioxidant in the body, dealing with the free radical damage.[4] Any wound in the body has plenty of free radicals because the immune cells use these highly reactive molecules for destroying microbes and toxins. Excess free radicals have to be neutralised, and cholesterol is one of the natural substances that accomplishes this function.[58]

When we have surgery, our tissues are cut and many small arteries, veins and capillaries get damaged. The liver receives a very strong signal from this damage, so it floods the body with LDL cholesterol to clean and heal every little wound in our blood vessels. That is why blood cholesterol goes high after any surgery.[31] After dental treatment, in addition to the damage to the tissues, a lot of bacteria from the tooth and the gums finish up in the blood, attacking the inside walls of our blood vessels. The liver gets a strong signal from that damage and produces lots of healing cholesterol to deal with it, so the blood cholesterol goes up.[32] The same thing happens when we have an infection – LDL cholesterol goes up to deal with the bacterial or viral attack.[54,56] Apart from the endothelium, our immune cells need cholesterol to function and to heal themselves after the fight with the infection.[56] Our stress hormones are made out of cholesterol in the body. Stressful situations increase our blood cholesterol levels because cholesterol is being sent to the adrenal glands for stress hormone production.[31] Apart from that, when we are under stress there is a storm of free radicals and other damaging biochemistry in the blood. So the liver works hard to produce and send out as much cholesterol as possible to deal with the free radical attack.[58] So again your blood cholesterol will test high.

In short, when we have a high blood cholesterol level it means that the body is dealing with some damage. The last thing we should do is interfere with this process! When the damage has been dealt with the blood cholesterol will naturally go down.[61] If we have an ongoing disease in the body that constantly inflicts damage, then the blood cholesterol will be permanently high.[49] So, when a doctor finds high cholesterol in a patient, what this doctor should do is to look for the reason. The doctor should ask, "What is damaging the body, so the liver has to produce all that cholesterol to deal with the damage?"

Unfortunately, instead of that, our doctors are trained to attack the cholesterol.

Many natural herbs, antioxidants and vitamins have an ability to reduce our blood cholesterol.[7,32,62] How do they do that? By helping the body to remove the damaging agents: be they free radicals, bacteria, viruses or toxins. As a result the liver does not have to produce so much cholesterol to deal with the damage. At the same time vitamins, minerals, antioxidants, herbs and other natural remedies help to heal the wound.[63] When the wound heals there is no need for the presence of cholesterol anymore, so the body removes it in the form of HDL cholesterol or so-called "good" cholesterol. That is why herbs, vitamins, antioxidants and other natural remedies increase the level of HDL cholesterol in the blood.[62,63]

In conclusion: cholesterol is one of the most essential substances in the body. We cannot live without it, let alone function well. The pernicious diet-heart hypothesis has vilified this essential substance. Unfortunately, this hypothesis has served many commercial and political interests far too well, so they ensure its long survival. However, the life of the diet-heart hypothesis is coming to an end as we become aware that cholesterol has been mistakenly blamed for the crime, just because it was found at the site of it. The "crime" is atherosclerosis. In the next chapter we are going to see exactly what atherosclerosis is, how it develops and what role cholesterol and fats play in its development.

Part Two: WHAT IS ATHEROSCLEROSIS?
Atherosclerosis is an inflammatory condition

From the very beginning to the very end formation of every athero-sclerotic plaque in your blood vessels is inflammation.[1,2,3,4,5] The universal marker for an ongoing inflammation in the body, called C-reactive protein, is rapidly becoming accepted as the best marker for atherosclerosis and for predicting its deadly complications: heart attacks and strokes.[6,7,8,9] Let us understand what this all means.

What is inflammation? It is a normal way for our bodies to respond to an injury. Imagine that one day some villain with a sledgehammer starts smashing your house. What are you going to do first – start repairing your house or try to deal with the villain? Of course, you are going to try and stop the villain first. You will call the police, your neighbours, your friends and together you will arrest the villain and remove him from the scene. Only then will you look at the damage and start repairs. The same thing happens in the body. Before any repair can start, the "villain", which is causing the injury, has to be destroyed and removed, and that is what inflammation does.

We are all familiar with **inflammation**. When we injure ourselves or have an infected wound the place becomes hot, painful, red and swollen. This is inflammation.[10] The injured cells release a whole group of chemicals (histamine, prostaglandins, leukotrienes, comple-ment, kinins and others), which send a message to the white blood cells, our "body police", to come and deal with the "villain".[11,12,13] At the same time they stimulate production of various proteins, such as fibrin, which wall off the damaged area, so the damage does not spread.[13] The white blood cells arrive and destroy the invader. In order to remove it from the scene a particular group of white blood cells, called phagocytes and macrophages, "swallow up" all the debris of the "villain" and the damaged tissues, "digest" them and remove them from the area.[12] When the site of the injury is "clean" the inflamma-tion gradually stops and gives way to repair.[14]

The **process of repair** involves the growth of so-called granulation tissue, made out of collagen, local cells, other repair materials and cholesterol.[15] Collagen is the most common protein in the body (about a third of all our body protein is collagen).[16] It is strong and flexible and, in a way, holds our tissues and organs together. Any repair process involves the growth of collagen fibres through the damaged tissue. Cholesterol is a healing agent in the body.[17,18] Together with collagen, it is an integral part of any scar tissue in any wound after it has been repaired.[19] As the repair proceeds new blood vessels grow through the repaired tissue, initially giving the scar a bright red colour. As collagen accumulates and constricts the newly grown blood vessels, the scar becomes tougher and whiter in colour.[10] That is when the repair process is complete.

This is what happens in a healthy body when an injury is inflicted upon any tissue or any organ. This is how Mother Nature has designed it: the inflammation and the repair, like two partners, work together in harmony.

However, in a growing number of the Western population this normal process goes wrong, leading to a disease, called **atherosclerosis**, or the formation of never-healing lesions, called atherosclerotic plaques, on the inside walls of blood vessels. A person may develop many plaques at the same time.[15] People commonly think that an **atherosclerotic plaque** is a lump of fat and cholesterol stuck to the wall of the artery. This simplistic idea is wrong. An atherosclerotic plaque is like an ulcer, erosion on the inside wall of the artery, covered by a mixture of debris, calcium, fibrin, foam cells, sclerotic tissue and chemically damaged fats.[20,21] The average composition of an advanced atherosclerotic plaque is as follows: 68% fibrous tissue (tissue of repair mainly made out of collagen), 8% calcium, 7% inflammatory cells, 1% foam cells and 16% lipid-rich necrotic core.[22] And the interesting fact is that in that lipid (fatty) part of the plaque most fats are unsaturated – 74% of total fatty acids.[23] According to the mainstream propaganda it is the 'deadly' saturated fat that is supposed to accumulate in the atherosclerotic plaque. Clearly the reality is very different: it is largely the unsaturated fats that accumulate in the plaque, and it is likely that they have come from the vegetable oils and cooking oils in the food.

The development of an atherosclerotic plaque is an out-of-order attempt by the body to deal with an injury inside our blood vessels. Accumulated research in the last few decades has established that the whole process is a runaway, out-of-control inflammation. Let us have a look at how it all happens.

Our vascular system is the transport network in our bodies, our motorway system if you will. Whatever damaging agents we have in our bodies, whether they are produced by our own tissues or got in from the outside, sooner or later finish up in the bloodstream.[15] These may be microbes, parasites, free radicals, various toxic substances, drugs, trans fatty acids, etc. While they are moving through our blood vessels they are going to attack. What are they going to attack first? Whatever is close – the inner lining of the blood vessels.[15] This is a thin layer of cells called **the endothelium**. Normal, healthy endothelium does not allow any blood cells to attach themselves to it. However, an injured endothelium immediately "calls" white blood cells to it and inflammation begins.[24,25] In a healthy situation everything goes according to Nature's plan: inflammation gets rid of the "villain", the repair process heals the damage and your artery is left as good as new. Unfortunately, in atherosclerosis we do not have a straightforward inflammation. It is a chronic, festering, never-ending inflammation, which competes with the process of repair. Sometimes the repair wins for a while, but then inflammation catches on and destroys the newly formed repair tissue in the arterial wall.[20]

In the following chapters we will try to understand why it all happens. But first let us see how it happens.

The formation of an atherosclerotic plaque has three stages.[26]

Stage one. A damaging agent in the bloodstream attacks the endothelium. Injury to the endothelium attracts white blood cells, which invade the site of the injury and go underneath the endothelium into deeper layers of the vascular wall.[27,28] Like soldiers in an army, their function is to destroy the damaging agent and clean the site. Cells, called macrophages, swallow the debris of damaged tissue, microbes, toxins and chemically damaged fats and swell to a large size. Now they are called foam cells.[28] White blood cells start multiplying at the site of the injury and new ones arrive from the blood stream to deal with the "villain" that caused the injury. This is inflammation in full flow.[29]

Stage two. While the inflammation is tearing things apart the process of repair starts. Arteries have muscular walls. These artery muscles are made out of so-called smooth muscle cells. These cells are considered to be the agents of repair.[30] They grow through the whole plaque and deeper into the wall of the blood vessel, making the plaque more permanent and well established. As the body tries to repair the damage, it stimulates the growth of collagen fibres through the plaque. The collagen forms a fibrous cap on top of the plaque, sealing it off.[31] When the inflammation stops and the repair process takes over, the plaque becomes sclerotic and calcium may settle in it. In effect, it is a scar inside your artery, which forms after the injury has been repaired.[31,32] If the size of this scar is small it may remain in the blood vessel without doing any harm. We all have these scars in our blood vessels, and the older we become the more of them we accumulate. If these scars are extensive, they may disfigure and narrow the artery and interfere with the blood flow.[32,33]

Unfortunately, in atherosclerosis the inflammation does not stop; it goes on and on. The repair and the inflammation continue alongside each other, which makes the plaque grow bigger.[20,26] It may grow slower or faster, depending on who is winning – the inflammation or the repair.[20] If, at any stage, the plaque occupies half of the vessel lumen or more, then it may partially obstruct the blood flow, causing various symptoms such as poor circulation in arms and legs (peripheral arterial disease); reduced blood flow to the brain, which can lead to poor memory, cognitive and neurological problems; damage to kidneys, leading to high blood pressure; and many other chronic symptoms, depending on which organ is affected.[34,35,36,37,38] If the coronary arteries, which feed the heart, are affected, the person will suffer from angina – severe chest pains caused by the lack of blood supply to the heart muscle.[39]

The muscular walls of the arteries can contract or relax. Various influences in the body can cause a spasm of the arteries.[40,41] If the artery is already half obstructed by an atherosclerotic plaque, then the spasm may close it up altogether.[40] Depending on how long the spasm lasts, the tissues, which this artery feeds, will starve. If it is an area of the brain, the person will suffer a transient stroke.[42] If the spasm is short, then the stroke may be mild; if the spasm lasts longer, then the damage from the stroke may be more serious. If the spasm happens in the coronary arteries, the heart muscle will starve. Because spasms are usually short lived they may not cause a heart attack, but they will damage a part of the heart tissues, leading to abnormalities in the heart beat, called arrhythmia.[37,43] Unfortunately, in some cases, the spasm is long enough to cause serious damage to the heart muscle and sudden death.[44]

This second stage of plaque development can last for many years. Depending on what is winning at the time – repair or inflammation – the plaque may become smaller or bigger.[20] At this stage the progression of an atherosclerotic plaque will stop only if the inflammation stops.[26] If the repair wins, the artery wall will heal without you ever knowing that you had a plaque there. If the inflammation continues or is rekindled after a period of time, the plaque progresses to its final third stage.[22,26]

Stage three. If inflammation persists, the plaque accumulates a crumbly, fatty core made out of dead white blood cells, debris of tissue, toxins and oxidised, chemically changed fats and cholesterol.[22,26] This core is similar to an accumulation of pus in an infected wound – an abscess. If an abscess is not drained it will erode surrounding tissues and burst. In the same way, ongoing inflammation in the atherosclerotic plaque stimulates production of certain enzymes, called collagenases, which start dissolving collagen.[22] As the fibrous cap on top of the plaque is largely made out of collagen, it becomes thin and weak and eventually ruptures.[26] This event is akin to a volcano exploding inside an artery. In a matter of seconds the blood coagulates, causing thrombosis, and the artery gets blocked.[45] This leads to the most dramatic and deadly complications of atherosclerosis – the heart attack and the stroke.

The "volcano explosion" produces certain chemicals (thromboxane A2, thrombin, serotonin and other thrombosis-associated mediators of vasoconstriction), which cause a prolonged spasm in the artery wall, not only at the site of the plaque but also anywhere downstream.[22,45] If the artery is wide enough not to get blocked at the site of the plaque, this spasm may close up smaller blood vessels downstream and cause heart attack or stroke in the area fed by these small arteries.[45,46] Apart from that a fragment of the plaque can break off and float downstream, blocking an artery, with the same consequences.[47]

Often all three things happen at the same time: the artery gets blocked at the site of the ruptured plaque, smaller vessels downstream go into a spasm and fragments of "burst" atherosclerotic plaque float downstream and block smaller arteries.[45,46,47] The result is starvation and death for the tissues normally fed by these arteries. Apart from the heart and the brain any organ and tissue in the body can be affected.

The plaque rupture and following thrombosis are the most devastating consequences of atherosclerosis. They cause approximately 76% of all fatal heart attacks.[15] This is what makes atherosclerosis a number one killer amongst all the diseases in the developed world. If these stage three, rupture-prone plaques could be prevented, atherosclerosis would be a much more benign disease.

What is special about these unstable plaques? Their core: like an abscess filled with pus, these plaques are filled with a crumbly, fatty, soft core containing virtually no cells, collagen or blood vessels. The bigger the core, the more unstable the plaque.[22,45,46,47] Because this core contains chemically damaged cholesterol, oxidised lipoproteins and other oxidised lipids they received the entire blame for heart attacks, strokes and other complications of atherosclerosis. If you are found at the site of the crime, you are likely to be blamed for it. However, recent advances in basic sciences have shown us that this blame is absolutely wrong.

Let us have a look at this core and try to understand what cholesterol and fats are really doing there.

It is an established scientific fact that the body uses fats and cholesterol as raw materials for building cells and tissues, which include all healing processes.[48,49,50] Let us see what the body uses these fats and cholesterol for at the site of the inflammation.

All cells in the body are largely made out of membranes. The cellular wall, the walls of organelles inside the cells and the walls that separate different compartments of the cell from each other are all membranes.[51] The membranes hold the cell together; without them the watery contents of the cell would just be a puddle on the floor. Our bodies are made out of cells; every organ, every tissue, every little speck of us is made out of cells. It has been estimated that from 40 to 80% of our body cells are membranes.[52] Based on that, we can estimate that a large percentage of our bodies is made out of those membranes. Well, what are the membranes made of?

The answer is this: all membranes are made out of fats and cholesterol, which means that our bodies are largely made out of fats and cholesterol![10,23]

Cholesterol is an essential part of any cell membrane; in fact, in many cells of the body almost half of the cell wall is made out of cholesterol.[18,23] The fats in the membranes are called phospholipids, which in turn are made out of one molecule of glycerol and two molecules of fatty acids: usually one saturated and one unsaturated.[53] At least half of the fatty acid part of the phospholipids are saturated fats because they, together with cholesterol, give the cell its stability and shape and allow it to fulfil its many functions.[23,53] Different kinds of cells in the body need different amounts of cholesterol and saturated fats, depending on what their function and purpose is.[52,53] These are scientific facts, which the majority of people are not aware of. Instead they are being brainwashed to believe that cholesterol and saturated fatty acids are the worst things on earth, when their bodies to a large degree are made out of these substances.

During the inflammation and repair of any tissue millions of new cells are born, each of which requires lots of cholesterol, phospholipids, saturated fats and other lipids for its membranes, structure and function. The repair of the vascular wall in atherosclerosis is no exception: new smooth muscle cells, white blood cells, macrophages and endothelial cells all need cholesterol, saturated fats and other lipids in order to be born in the first place and then to function.[54,55,59] White blood cells rely on cholesterol in fighting an infection and repairing themselves after a fight.[56] Inflammation is a fight, which employs millions of white blood cells as its "soldiers". So, inflammation always requires a lot of cholesterol, saturated fats and other lipids as building materials for creating its "soldiers" and as a repair agent for the "wounded" ones.[18,20] Every site of inflammation gives out a "call" for fats and cholesterol, which is normally received by the liver.[23] The liver gets into gear and starts producing lots of various fats and cholesterol, packaging them into shuttles called lipoproteins and sending them to the place of inflammation.[57,58]

Lipoproteins are like little bags made out of protein and lipids: they are water-soluble on the outside and fat-soluble on the inside.[52,53] Cholesterol, fats, steroids, fat-soluble vitamins and many other molecules in the body are fat-soluble; they cannot travel in the water-based blood without being packaged into lipoproteins. A lot of toxins and drugs are also fat-soluble and travel through the body inside lipoproteins.[52,53] The body makes many different lipoproteins. The cholesterol produced in the liver is sent to the site of inflammation in a lipoprotein called LDL (low-density lipoprotein). That is why a person with active inflammation in the body will always have high levels of blood LDL cholesterol. Triglycerides (another variety of fat produced in the liver) are packaged into a VLDL (very low-density lipoprotein) and sent to the site of inflammation to be used for building the cell structure, defence from infection and energy production.[23,52,53] Other fats, vital for repair, also get sent to the site of damage inside lipoproteins. They will keep arriving until they are not needed any more. In the case of atherosclerosis the inflammation never stops, so the need for cholesterol, phospholipids, saturated fats, triglycerides and other fats never stops either.[60,61,62,63]

The problem is that the site of inflammation has an ability to damage and chemically change these healing fats and cholesterol.[59] There are different ways to inflict this damage, but the one we know most about is free-radical damage. Let us see how it happens.

n the process of inflammation a lot of free radicals are created.[64,65,66] Free radicals are very reactive molecules which, if let loose, can cause a lot of damage to anything in sight.[23,64] There is a good reason why they are there: the white blood cells (the soldiers) use free radicals as "missiles and bullets" in killing the infectious agents and dealing with toxins. The site of inflammation is like a battlefield with lots of bullets and missiles flying everywhere. The excess free radicals have to be neutralised. The substances that accomplish this function are called antioxidants.[10]

Antioxidants are also an essential part of any inflammation and repair process in the body.[52] The body makes many antioxidants to deal with excess free radicals, and one of these antioxidants is cholesterol.[48,68] Unfortunately, like all antioxidants, as cholesterol quenches the free radicals it gets damaged itself. To rescue this damaged cholesterol the liver sends another lipoprotein, called HDL (high-density lipoprotein).[53,58] HDL carries other antioxidants to the site of the inflammation, rescues cholesterol and carries it back to the liver to be recycled. Fats are particularly prone to free radical damage.[23] If they are not protected by antioxidants, fats get damaged quite quickly in inflamed tissues. In a healthy body this damage can be reversed by other antioxidants: vitamin C, vitamin E, other vitamins, carotenoids, lipoic acid and other nutrients. It has been demonstrated in clinical experiments that supplementing high doses of antioxidants reduces the size of atherosclerotic plaques, sometimes quite dramatically.[67,68,70] For example, supplementing high doses of vitamin C alone can be so successful in treating atherosclerosis, that some researchers consider the disease to be nothing more than a low-grade scurvy.[69,70,71] Unfortunately, in our modern world with our modern processed diets, the majority of people are deficient in antioxidants.[58] So, damaged cholesterol and damaged fats don't get a chance to be rescued and removed from the "battlefield"; instead they either get swallowed by the foam cells or just deposited in the middle of the plaque.[34,36,37] On top of that our modern diet provides a lot of processed fats, full of oxidised and chemically damaged lipids and cholesterol. The body cannot use these substances so they too finish up being swallowed by the foam cells and deposited in the plaque.[72,73,74]

These chemically damaged fats, lipoproteins and cholesterol cannot be used by the body for producing new cells, healing, repair or anything else. Like disposed garbage they just accumulate in the "battlefield", filling up the crumbly core of the atherosclerotic plaque, together with the debris of dead cells, broken-down collagen, burst foam cells and other destroyed tissues.[75] As the repair tries to build new collagen, new cells and new blood vessels, the inflammation destroys them, turning them all into dead necrotic debris. In an atherosclerotic plaque inflammation and repair go on alongside each other, competing with each other. As both the inflammation and the repair need lots of cholesterol and fats, the body keeps delivering these substances to the site of the plaque until either repair wins (and turns the plaque into a sclerotic scar) or the inflammation wins. If the inflammation wins, it takes the plaque to its catastrophic, final, third stage.[26]

As we can see, cholesterol, saturated fats, lipoproteins and other fats do not cause atherosclerosis. They are just victims of the out-of-control inflammation going on in the plaque. They get slaughtered, together with white blood cells, endothelial cells, collagen, newly formed blood vessels and other molecules and structures. All these destroyed dead things form the crumbly core of the plaque, and the bigger this core becomes, the more unstable and dangerous the plaque becomes.

In this chapter we have discussed **how** atherosclerosis develops.

However, it doesn't have to develop at all!

What we must understand is that an atherosclerotic plaque is not cast in stone. At any stage in its development the plaque can be reduced in size, removed altogether or keep progressing and growing. The fate of the plaque depends entirely on what is happening in the body biochemically.[76] The human body has excellent mechanisms to prevent the formation of these plaques altogether or to dissolve and remove them. That is, if it is allowed to do so! Unfortunately, our modern lifestyles do not allow our bodies to look after themselves.

In the next chapter we are going to examine **why** atherosclerosis develops. We will look at the factors that create a perfect environment in the body for plaque formation and its progression to its final catastrophic stage, leading to heart attacks, strokes and other complications. We will try to understand what we are doing wrong to create this number one killer-disease in our very sophisticated, developed world. We have been barking up the wrong tree for a long time, thanks to the faulty diet-heart hypothesis. Now we know that atherosclerosis is not caused by dietary fats and cholesterol, it is caused by chronic out-of-control inflammation. So, let us see why we have this inflammation and why it gets out of control.

What causes atherosclerosis?

All our blood vessels – arteries, veins and capillaries, as well as our heart, on their inside walls are covered with a thin layer of cells, called **endothelium**.[1,2] This layer of cells separates the flowing blood from the rest of the body, and if its total mass could be laid flat it would cover a very large area.[1] The more we learn about the endothelium the more amazed we become at how complex and magnificent this thin layer of cells is! It is an organ in itself, accomplishing a myriad of functions. It is a major player in the communication between our blood (and anything in the blood) and the rest of the body.[1,2,3] It controls blood coagulation, producing both pro-thrombotic (making the blood clot) and anti-thrombotic substances, as well as fibrinolitics (which dissolve blood clots) and anti-fibrinolitics.[1,3] It controls the muscle tone of the walls of the blood vessels and the heart, telling them to contract or relax, which makes their lumen (the space inside) wider or narrower.[1,2,3] It produces many hormones (autocrine, paracrine and endocrine) to communicate with local cells, nearby tissues and the rest of the body. In fact, endothelium is now considered to be the biggest and most important endocrine gland we have.[4,5,6] It controls a fine balance of electrolytes and other chemical substances in the tissues, which makes it one of the major regulators of our homeostasis (the finely tuned balance in the body).[4,5] It responds immediately to any chemical or physical agent in the blood and "reports" it to the rest of the body, so the body can adjust straight away. It regulates our blood pressure, our blood sugar, our blood electrolytes and many other parameters.[1,2,4] It controls the state of the blood cells and surrounding tissue cells, playing a part in their appropriate growth, maturation and movement. It is a major regulator of immune responses in the body, orchestrating the behaviour of white blood cells and other aspects of immunity.[4,5,6] But one of its most important functions is response to any injury we sustain: endothelium is a major player in inflammation and repair in the body.[1,4,7,8]

So, what attacks and injures endothelium? What initiates inflammation in our blood vessels? What kind of influences are we talking about?

The list is long and is getting longer. Anything harmful we allow into our bodies gets into the bloodstream quite quickly. Once in the bloodstream, these substances attack your endothelium.

Let us start with things close to home, things we expose ourselves to every single day.

- Man-made chemicals. Every time you use personal care products you cause endothelial injury.[9] For a long time we thought that skin was a barrier, which did not let things through. Now we know better – our skin absorbs most things we put on it almost instantly.[10,11,12,13,14] The pharmaceutical industry has become aware of this fact and is producing more and more drugs in the form of patches and creams.[12,13] When we swallow the drug as a pill, before it absorbs and goes into the bloodstream, it has to go through the liver, which will destroy most of the drug. By applying the drug to the skin, it enters your bloodstream in seconds, without having to pass the test of the liver.[11,13] Personal care products (toothpaste, shampoos, bubble baths, shower gels, makeup, perfumes, deodorants, hair dyes and other lotions and potions) are made out of man-made chemicals, most of which are toxic and have been proven to cause cancer and many other health problems.[10,13,14,15,16] They absorb through skin in seconds and finish up in your bloodstream, attacking your endothelium and the rest of the body. We have been systematically seduced into using more and more of these toxic things, which we do not need. We humans lived perfectly well without them for millennia. It is important to avoid most personal care products if we want to avoid heart disease, cancer and many other degenerative diseases. For those few personal care products you *really* need you can find many natural, non-toxic alternatives on the market.
- More man-made chemicals. People who are very house proud, who use a lot of domestic cleaning chemicals and frequently redecorate their houses, expose themselves to hundreds of toxic chemicals.[11,16] They absorb quickly through our skin and lungs into the bloodstream and cause endothelial injury and dysfunction.[10,13,16] It is very important to remove these toxins from your family's life and replace them with natural alternatives.

- More man-made chemicals. Laundry and dish-washer detergents are toxic and do not rinse off your clothes, bedding, towels, your dishes, cutlery and kitchen utensils. As a result, you allow hundreds of toxins into your body through your skin and your digestive system.[10,11,12,14,16] Most laundry detergents are highly perfumed, so you breathe in toxic chemicals from your clothes day in and day out. All these chemicals finish up in your blood and will attack your endothelium and the rest of the body. Thankfully, today there are natural, non perfumed alternatives available on the market.

- More man-made chemicals. Prescription and over-the-counter drugs are all toxins.[10,11,12,13] Apart from the active ingredient, the drug will have dozens of other ingredients, many of which have been proven to cause cancer, heart disease and other health problems: preservatives, fillers, binders, colours, emulsifiers, etc. Dr Samuel Epstein, MD, in his book *Unreasonable Risk* states: "A recent survey of 241 high-volume US prescription drugs reported that nearly half posed cancer risks based on carcinogenicity tests designed by industry, or government to prove safety... prescription drugs may pose the single most important class of unrecognised and avoidable carcinogenic risks for the entire US population".[10] Anything that can cause cancer would cause endothelial injury and atherosclerosis. Drugs, which are taken on a long-term basis are the most dangerous ones. The Western population is consuming staggering amounts of various drugs.[17] Taking pills has become so common that people do not question, or even think about what these drugs are doing to them.

- Smokers, and those of us who are too polite to stop a selfish smoker from turning us into passive smokers, expose themselves to a plethora of chemicals and free radicals, which injure their endothelium and start atherosclerotic process in their blood vessels.[18,19]

- Industrial pollution. Hundreds of studies from all over the world have demonstrated that living in an industrial polluted area near factories, waste incinerators, airports, big roads and other polluters dramatically increases morbidity and mortality from heart disease.[20,21,22,23] Industrial pollution will expose you to large amounts of man-made chemicals, which will get into your bloodstream and cause endothelial injury and atherosclerosis.

- Pesticides, herbicides, chemical fertilisers and other agricultural chemicals in our food and water end up in our blood and cause endothelial injury and dysfunction.[10,11,24] It is important to eat only organic and ecologically clean food if we want to prevent disease.
- Chlorine, fluoride, nitrates and other contaminants in our drinking water cause atherosclerosis.[10,11] It is a good idea to filter your drinking water. Avoid fluoride in water, toothpaste and anything else; it is extremely poisonous. (There is a lot of information on fluoride available, if you look for it.)[25] Avoid the toxic, chlorinated "soup" of swimming pools![15] Nature has designed us to swim in the natural waters of seas, oceans, lakes and rivers, which are health-giving.
- Processed foods, which are generally nutritionally empty and full of added chemicals, cause endothelial injury.[26,27] These foods are full of chemically altered proteins and carbohydrates, damaging trans fats and other chemically mutilated fats, other destroyed nutrients and added man-made chemicals, such as flavourings, preservatives, E numbers, etc.[26,27,28,29] Processed foods do not feed our bodies; they pollute and damage them. It is vital to avoid these foods in order to prevent atherosclerosis and heart disease.
- Various infectious microbes, getting into the bloodstream, will attack the endothelium and start an inflammatory process. Many different infectious organisms have been found in human atherosclerotic plaques: *Chlamydia pneumoniae, Helicobacter pylori, Cytomegalovirus, Herpes zoster virus* and *Bacteroides gingivalis* among them.[30,31,32,33,34,35,36] These microbes generally get into the bloodstream from any site of chronic infection in the body: the stomach and the rest of the digestive system, infected gums and teeth, infected sinuses, infected skin and other infected organs. The very fact that these infections survive in the body, let alone get into the bloodstream, means that the immune system is not in good shape. Normally the human body has excellent mechanisms for dealing with infections. However, all the factors we have already discussed will weaken our defences and allow infections to thrive.
- Abnormalities in gut flora will flood the body with a plethora of toxins and dangerous microbes. Gut flora is a mass of microbes which live inside our digestive systems. Gut flora is an essential part

of our human physiology and, in a healthy person, is dominated by beneficial health-giving microbes.[37] Overuse of antibiotics and other drugs have damaged gut flora in a large percentage of the Western population, causing a condition called gut dysbiosis.[38] In this situation disease-causing microbes replace the beneficial ones. They upset the digestive process and damage the gut lining, which allows all sorts of toxins and pathogenic microbes to get into the bloodstream.[39,40] If you want proof, find a practitioner who can do live blood microscopy for you, and see for yourself what kind of creatures float in your blood vessels. Once in the blood these microbes injure the endothelium and start the atherosclerotic process.[41,42] It is very important to look after your digestive system and its gut flora (more on this subject later).

- Nutritional deficiencies in many vitamins, minerals, amino acids, essential fats and other nutrients will cause endothelial damage.[44,51] The endothelium constantly renews itself and heals any injuries that it sustains from man-made chemicals, microbes, free radicals, trans fats, processed foods, toxins and anything else.[43,44,45] In order to repair itself, it needs nutrients: amino acids, vitamins, minerals, fats, etc. Our modern diets do not provide many of these nutrients, and as a result do not allow the endothelium to look after itself. Literally every few months new scientific studies come out, showing how supplementing different vitamins, amino acids, oils, minerals, herbs and other nutrients reverses atherosclerotic process.[46,51,52] They reverse it because they allow the endothelium to heal itself. Nutritional deficiencies also upset biochemistry in the body, creating many harmful substances that damage endothelium. One example of such harmful substances is an amino acid called homocysteine, which causes injury, inflammation and plaque formation in the endothelium.[47,48,49] It appears in the body when we are deficient in vitamins B6, B12 and folate; supplementing these vitamins stops production of homocysteine in the body. Another example is a substance, called Lp(a) or Lipoprotein(a), which is a sign of vitamin C deficiency.[49,50] People with high levels of Lp(a) are almost 70% more likely to have a heart attack.[50] All we have to do to remove this risk is consume plenty of organic fresh and fermented vegetables and fruit, which will provide our bodies with vitamin C.

- Lack of sun exposure does not allow the endothelium to heal itself after any injury. When we sunbathe, vitamin D – the sunshine vitamin – is produced in our skin. It is a vitamin no cell, no tissue and no organ in our bodies can live without, let alone repair itself after an injury.[53,54] Recent misguided fear of sun has caused an epidemic of vitamin D deficiency in the Western world. This deficiency is now one of the recognised causes of the heart disease epidemic.[55,56] There is no connection between skin cancer and sun exposure, as far as solid science is concerned.[55,57,58,59,60,61,62,63,64,65] However, commercial powers that profit from sunscreen lotion sales have launched a multibillion propaganda, which unfortunately has influenced the medical profession as well.[66] This propaganda has created sun phobia in the population. Incidentally, many sunscreen lotions contain chemicals that have been proven to cause skin cancer.[63,64,65,66] Just exposing your face and hands to the sun is not enough to produce significant amounts of vitamin D; you need to expose your whole body. That is why sensible sunbathing is not only natural for us, humans, but absolutely essential. Lack of sun exposure, and hence vitamin D deficiency, is the explanation for the fact that people with darker skin, who move to colder countries, are particularly prone to atherosclerosis and its deadly complications – the so-called South Asian paradox in the UK.[67,68] The pigmentation in dark-skinned people does not allow enough sunlight through, essential for vitamin D production.[68,69,70] When dark-skinned people live in countries with lots of strong sunlight, they do not have this problem. However, when they move to colder countries with much lower sun exposure, they put themselves at risk. So, taking any opportunity to sunbathe is particularly important for dark-skinned people.
- A sedentary lifestyle,[72] excessive stress,[71] free radicals,[45] electromagnetic pollution,[73] radiation[74] and other influences can all cause endothelial injury and development of atherosclerosis.[71]

In our modern world we are often exposed to many of these influences at once. They all injure our endothelium and start an inflammatory process within it.[71] However, these influences only represent half of the story. Under normal conditions, after any injury the endothelium would go through inflammation, then repair and be done with it.

However, in the development of atherosclerosis, inflammation never stops. Why does it never stop? Because we have another major factor in our modern world that does not allow it to stop.

Let me introduce you to the main villain in the development of atherosclerosis and its deadly complications. It is called Metabolic Syndrome.

What is metabolic syndrome?

Metabolic syndrome is a situation where your blood is full of sugar (called glucose) and full of hormone insulin (hyperinsulinemia). It is an extremely common condition, due to our modern eating habits, and in many cases it starts developing in childhood.[75]

Blood glucose, or blood sugar, is normally kept within certain strict limits by the body, because too high or too low will lead to hundreds of health complications including death.[4] The body has solid mechanisms for controlling blood sugar level. The most important is a hormone, called insulin, produced by your pancreas. After any meal carbohydrates absorb as molecules of glucose and raise your blood glucose (blood sugar) level. Glucose cannot leave your bloodstream and enter the tissues and organs of your body without the help of insulin; insulin is the key that opens the "doors" on the cell walls of your organs and lets the glucose in. Once in the cell glucose is used for producing energy, building cellular structure and other functions. Insulin converts any excessive glucose into fat and stores it in your fat tissues for a rainy day. When the blood sugar goes down to a normal level, the production of insulin stops and the blood level also goes down to normal. That is what happens in a healthy, normal situation.[75,76,77,78]

However, we have created a very abnormal and unhealthy situation in our modern world of plenty. We have created **processed carbohydrates!**

What are processed carbohydrates? All those breakfast cereals, crisps, biscuits, crackers, breads, cakes, ice creams, pastries, pastas, chocolates, sweets, popcorn, jams, condiments, sugar and anything that contains it, preserved fruit and vegetables, soft drinks (sodas and pops) and beer, processed fruit juices and frozen precooked meals with starches and batter are processed carbohydrates.

All carbohydrates in foods get digested and absorbed largely as molecules of glucose. Nature provides us with plenty of carbohydrates in the form of fruit, vegetables, seeds and grains. When we eat them in their natural, unprocessed form, the carbohydrate gets absorbed slowly, producing a gradual increase in blood glucose, which our bodies are designed to handle.[78,79] Also the carbohydrate part of whole natural foods does not all get absorbed; in fact, a large part of it is indigestible for us, humans, which limits the amount of glucose molecules entering the bloodstream.[79]

Processed carbohydrates are created in our big factories where natural foods are subjected to heavy processing. As a result processed carbohydrates are very easy to digest. They get absorbed almost fully, putting excessive amounts of glucose into our bloodstream, which our physiology has not been designed to handle. In addition, processed carbohydrates pile all that glucose in very quickly, producing an unnaturally rapid increase in blood glucose.[80] A person who has a breakfast cereal in the morning, a sandwich for lunch and pasta in the evening, with soft drinks, crisps, biscuits, pastries, sweets, ice cream, cakes, sugar and chocolate bars in between, loads their body with massive, unnatural amounts of glucose. If this situation happens rarely, the human body can manage it by storing all the excessive glucose as fat.[77] However, in our modern world, this situation happens daily from a very young age. Any substance, when put into the body in excess on a regular basis, will start destroying the body. The Western population is relentlessly gorging on huge amounts of glucose as if there is no tomorrow.

The normal physiological reaction to excessive carbohydrate is to store it as fat. So, we have an obesity epidemic.[81] Tragically not only adults but also children are the victims. Children in the Western world are becoming more and more obese because they consume processed carbohydrates just as much as adults do. A culture where sweets, crisps, ice cream, sweet drinks, cakes and biscuits are given to children as "treats" and snacks, floods their little bodies with massive amounts of glucose and starts a lifetime of metabolic syndrome and its deadly consequences: obesity, diabetes, atherosclerosis, heart disease and cancer.[76]

As we have already mentioned, it is insulin that brings down the blood sugar level. When glucose keeps pouring into the body in huge amounts, the person ends up with permanently high levels of insulin in their blood. This situation is called **hyperinsulinemia** (high insulin in the blood).[79] Remember, the role of insulin is to let glucose out of the blood into the cells of the body (your muscles, your brain, etc). However, our body cells have a limited capacity for taking in glucose. When there is too much glucose coming in and too much insulin to push that glucose into the cells, the cells just say, "Enough!" The way they say it is to destroy the "doors" on their cell walls, which insulin opens. That is how the cells in the body protect themselves from the glucose onslaught – they become insulin resistant. But the person keeps eating processed carbohydrates, so glucose keeps pouring in and its level in the blood becomes dangerously high. The body responds by producing more insulin to ram that glucose into the cells by force. The cells respond by becoming more insulin resistant. As a result, the pancreas produces even more insulin and hyperinsulinemia becomes more and more severe.[75,76,78,79] As insulin is our master fat-storage hormone, the person with permanently high levels of insulin in the blood can never lose weight; they just store most of their food as fat. Hyperinsulinemia is the cause of our obesity epidemic.[79,82] Obesity is just one thing that hyperinsulinemia will do to you; there are many more.

This is where we come back to our atherosclerosis and its deadly consequences – heart attacks and strokes. *Hyperinsulinemia creates a pro-inflammatory environment in the body.* It alters the biochemistry in such a way that inflammation is encouraged and cannot be terminated.[75,83,84,85] When we injure our endothelium, inflammation begins in the vascular wall, and because of hyperinsulinemia it cannot stop. The whole process is silent. It is the kind of quiet, insidious inflammation that we are not aware of. It sets off the whole process of the initiation and growth of atherosclerotic plaque, all the way to its fatal third stage, leading to a heart attack or a stroke.[86,87]

Metabolic syndrome is the basis for type 2 diabetes. That is why diabetics suffer from atherosclerosis and die from heart attacks and strokes more than anybody else.[83]

Having too much insulin in your bloodstream is one of the most dangerous things you can suffer from. The pro-inflammatory situation will not only set the scene for atherosclerosis, but also encourage many other degenerative conditions in your body: cancer, rheumatoid arthritis,

Alzheimer's disease, multiple sclerosis, other auto-immune conditions, inflammatory bowel disease, etc, etc.[78,79,87,83]

As all our hormones work as a team, abnormal levels of insulin in the body will get your other hormones out of balance: thyroid hormones, sex hormones and adrenal hormones.[79] These imbalances will lead to a myriad of symptoms, from low thyroid function, PMS, infertility, impotence and low immunity to depression, mood swings, sleep disorders and abnormal body shape.

We have talked about what excessive insulin will do to you. But what about all that excessive glucose in the blood? It does not sit there silently; it causes a lot of damage in its own right.

What can excessive blood sugar do to you?

The excess glucose in the bloodstream adds another major damaging factor to our list of damaging factors that injure the endothelium and cause lots of other damage in the body. Free molecules of glucose are very reactive; they attach themselves to proteins in the blood, making those proteins very sticky (the scientific name for these proteins is **AGEs – Advanced Glycosylated End products**).[88] These proteins stick to the walls of the blood vessels, damaging them and starting the atherosclerotic process.[89,90] Apart from that they get into small arteries and capillaries, block them and accumulate as a nasty substance called amyloid.[88,89,90] It commonly blocks capillaries in the retina of the eyes, causing poor eyesight and blindness.[91] Accumulating in the capillary bed of the kidneys it causes kidney problems and high blood pressure.[92,93] Accumulating in the capillaries of the brain it causes Alzheimer's disease.[94] Accumulating in the rich capillary bed of the male sexual organs it causes erectile dysfunction and impotence.[95] Wherever these AGEs accumulate, they cause serious problems. Diabetics have high levels of AGEs; hence they are very prone to blindness, kidney failure, impotence and loss of memory.[96,97,98] So, that spoonful of sugar is not as innocent as you may think!

Forming AGEs is not the only way glucose overload damages our bodies. It provides another factor that is a major contributor to heart disease, high blood pressure, and many other health problems. We are talking about **chronic magnesium deficiency.** Magnesium is a mineral that we cannot live without. It is involved in about 300 different metabolic reactions in the body.[77,79] Every cell, every tissue and every organ needs magnesium every second of your life. Unfortunately, our diet does not provide very much magnesium. It is mainly found in green leafy vegetables and nuts, which the majority of people do not eat much of; other foods contain magnesium in much smaller amounts.[80] Modern farming techniques strip the soils of magnesium, so food grown on these soils has very little of this mineral.[100] However, even our modern diets could perhaps provide enough, if we did not eat processed carbohydrates. As processed carbohydrates overload the body with glucose, they strip it of whatever precious magnesium the body has. Why? Because, in order to metabolise one molecule of glucose, we need at least 28 molecules of magnesium.[80,101] Like a swarm of locusts descending on a field and stripping it bare, the flood of glucose coming into the body leaves it severely deficient in magnesium (see the footnote).

On top of that, we add another common factor for magnesium deficiency – man-made chemicals. The body has wonderful mechanisms to deal with toxins, whether they are produced internally or come from outside. However, every detoxification pathway requires magnesium.[78,79,101] As we pollute ourselves with all sorts of chemicals, we create more magnesium deficiency in the body.

What happens to us when we are magnesium deficient?

A long list of problems:

- In order to contract our muscles need calcium; in order to relax they need magnesium. When we are magnesium deficient our muscles are unable to relax.[99,100] What does this mean for us? It means that you get high blood pressure because your arterial muscles cannot relax.[103,104] It means backache, neck pain and lumbago because the hundreds of muscles that support your spine go into a spasm.[99,102] It means cramps and eclampsia in pregnancy.[100,102] It means abnormalities in heart rhythm (arrhythmia) and sudden heart pains (angina pectoris).[102,104,105] It is the cause of sudden cardiac death because coronary arteries go into a spasm.[99,100,102] It is the cause of

---

Table sugar (sucrose) is made out of 2 molecules of mono-sugars (glucose and fructose), so it requires some 56 molecules of magnesium to be processed.

transient strokes as the brain arteries go into a spasm.[99,100] Any muscle in the body can go into a spasm with serious symptoms if you are deficient in magnesium: cramps, tremors, seizures, eye twitches, migraines, bronchial spasm, asthma, Raynaud's syndrome (the peripheral arteries go in a spasm, cutting blood supply), spastic colon, etc, etc.[99,100,102]

- Sudden death in athletes.[99,106] When athletes train they sweat; a lot of magnesium leaves the body through sweat.[80] If an athlete is already deficient in magnesium because of processed carbohydrates, and consumes so-called "energy" drinks, full of sugar, making him even more magnesium deficient, then his heart muscles can go into a spasm, leading to sudden death.
- Neurological and psychiatric symptoms: anxiety, depression, obsessions, hyperactivity, inability to concentrate, poor memory, vertigo, psychosis, confusion, panic attacks, aggression, mood disorders, etc.[107,108,109]
- Magnesium deficiency stimulates the release of histamine from the mast cells in the body. As a result the person becomes prone to allergies: hay fever, asthma, eczema, etc.[110]
- Hypokalemia, or low potassium in the body, is impossible to correct if the person is magnesium deficient.[110,111] Many drugs (such as diuretics, blood pressure pills and others) cause this condition, and no matter how much potassium you might take, you will suffer from hypokalemia until the magnesium is replenished. Many other deficiency conditions in the body also cannot be corrected if the body is deficient in magnesium.[111]
- Deficiency in magnesium will knock the rest of the minerals in the body out of balance and upset their functions: manganese, copper, zinc, molybdenum, iron and potassium.[99,100,111]
- Magnesium deficiency causes endothelial injury and dysfunction.[112,113]

If you speak to doctors who have tried to deal with magnesium deficiency in their patients, they will tell you just how difficult it is to correct! In fact, it is impossible to correct until the person stops eating processed carbohydrates. Due to consumption of these foods it is estimated that at least 80% of the Western population is chronically deficient in magnesium.[100,110]

In conclusion:

The modern world we have created exposes us to hundreds of influences, which injure our endothelium day in and day out. Normally the healing process of any injury goes through two stages:

1. inflammation,
2. repair.

Atherosclerosis and heart disease were virtually unknown until we invented processed carbohydrates. They create metabolic syndrome. Metabolic syndrome sets the scene in the body for perpetual inflammation. In that situation any injury to the endothelium cannot be healed. In a person who eats processed carbohydrates daily, the repair has to compete with relentless inflammation, leading to the formation of an unstable atherosclerotic plaque. As the plaque ruptures, it leads to a heart attack, a stroke or another disaster, depending on where in the body it happens. A considerable percentage of heart attacks and strokes happen due to the spasm of the artery – the result of severe magnesium deficiency, again caused by the consumption of processed carbohydrates and other processed foods. Apart from that, consumption of processed carbohydrates floods the body with too much glucose and creates AGEs (sticky proteins blocking up small blood vessels), causing Alzheimer's disease, kidney failure, vision loss and blindness (due to diabetic retinopathy or macular degeneration) and many other problems.

In this chapter we have discussed **why** atherosclerosis develops, what causes it and **why** it has become such an epidemic in our modern world. However, you do not have to become its victim! Most of the factors we have discussed here are under your personal control. With a few changes in your lifestyle you can prevent this scourge from touching you or your family.

In the next chapter we are going to see what we need to do to avoid falling prey to atherosclerosis and its complications, including heart attacks and strokes.

Part Three: WHAT TO DO?

What do we do to prevent atherosclerosis, heart attacks and strokes?

The answer is simple:

1. Stop eating processed foods!
2. Stop polluting your body with chemicals!

By accomplishing these two simple steps you will remove most of the risk. You will prevent falling prey not only to atherosclerosis and its complications but also to all the other degenerative diseases that plague the human race today, such as cancer, autoimmune conditions, memory loss, Alzheimer's disease, diabetes, etc.

Let us look at these two steps in more detail.

Step 1: Stop eating processed foods!

> *"Do you know what breakfast cereal is made of?
> It's made of all those little curly wooden shavings
> you find in pencil sharpeners!"*
>
> Roald Dahl,
> *Charlie and the Chocolate Factory*, 1964

We live in an era of convenience foods, which are very processed foods. When Mother Nature made our human bodies, she at the same time provided us with every food we need to stay healthy, active and full of energy. However, we have to eat these foods in the form that Nature made them. It is when we start tampering with natural foods that we start getting into trouble. Any processing that we subject the food to changes its chemical and biological structure. Our bodies were not designed to have these changed foods! The more food is processed, the more nutrient depleted and chemically altered it becomes.[1,2,4,5] Apart from losing its nutritional value, processed food loses most of its other properties: taste, flavour and colour. So, to compensate for that various chemicals are added: flavour enhancers, colours, various E numbers and other additives.[1,2,3,4,5] Many of these chemicals have been conclusively shown to contribute to inflammation, cancer, memory loss, hyperactivity and learning disabilities, psychiatric disorders and other health problems.[6,7,8,9,10,11] Natural foods do not keep very well, so industry changes them to prolong their shelf life. To achieve that natural foods are subjected to extreme heat, pressure, enzymes, solvents and countless numbers of various other chemicals; fats are hydrogenated, carbohydrates are modified and proteins are denatured.[1,2,3] In the process natural foods are changed into various chemical concoctions, which are then packaged nicely and presented to us as "food". "Food" that is made to suit commercial purposes where health considerations never enter the calculation. The manufacturers are obliged to list all the ingredients on the label. However, if the manufacturer uses an ingredient, that has already been processed or is made from processed substances, this manufacturer is not obliged to list what that ingredient was made from.[2,3] So, if you are trying to avoid something in particular, like sugar or gluten, for example, reading an ingredient list may not always help you.

If we look at supermarket shelves, we will see that the bulk of processed foods are carbohydrates. Breakfast cereals, crisps, soft drinks and beer, biscuits, crackers, breads, pastries, pastas, chocolates, sweets, jams, condiments, sugar, preserved fruit and vegetables, frozen precooked meals with starches and batter are all highly processed carbohydrates. In the previous chapter we talked about their role in setting the scene for perpetual inflammation and atherosclerosis. However, they have other immediate negative effects on the body.

Processed carbohydrates get absorbed very quickly, producing an unnaturally rapid increase in blood glucose.[12] A rapid increase in blood glucose, called **hyperglycaemia**, puts the body into a state of shock, prompting it to pump out lots of insulin very quickly to deal with the excessive glucose.[12,13] As a result of this overproduction of insulin, about an hour later the person has a very low level of blood glucose, called **hypoglycaemia**. Have any of you noticed that after eating a sugary breakfast cereal in the morning you feel hungry again in an hour? That is hypoglycaemia. What do people usually have at that time in the morning to satisfy their hunger? A biscuit, a chocolate bar, a coffee or something like that, and the whole cycle of hyper-hypoglycaemia begins again. This up and down blood glucose roller coaster is extremely harmful for anyone, children and adults alike. It has been proven that mood swings, lethargy, hyperactivity, inability to concentrate and learn, aggression and other behavioural abnormalities in children and adults are a direct result of this glucose roller coaster.[14,15,16,17] The hyperglycaemic phase produces the feeling of a "high", with hyperactive and manic tendencies, whilst the hypoglycaemic phase makes us feel unwell, often with a headache, bad mood, aggression and general fatigue.

Another important point about processed carbohydrates is their detrimental effect on the gut flora.[18,19] Processed carbohydrates feed pathogenic bacteria and fungi in the gut, promoting their growth and proliferation. Apart from that they make a wonderful glue-like environment in the gut for various worms and parasites to take hold and develop.[20,21] Many of these microbes and creatures produce toxic substances that go into the bloodstream and literally "poison" the person.[22,23] By negatively altering the gut flora, processed carbohydrates also play an important role in damaging the person's immune system because gut flora is a major regulator of the immune status. And, as if that is not enough processed foods (particularly processed carbohydrates and sugar) directly weaken the functioning of macrophages, natural killer cells and other immune cells, and undermine systemic resistance to all infections.[17,21,22,23,24] People who have sugary drinks, crisps, sweets, breakfast cereals and other processed foods daily worsen their immune system's condition by these food choices.

Let us have a look at some of the most common forms of processed carbohydrates.

Breakfast cereals

They are supposed to be healthy, aren't they? That is what numerous TV advertisements tell us. Unfortunately, the truth is just the opposite.[17,25,26]

- Breakfast cereals are highly processed carbohydrates, full of sugar, salt, trans fats and other unhealthy substances. A bowl of breakfast cereal will start your day with the first round of the blood sugar roller coaster, with its all too familiar symptoms for you to deal with.
- Being a great source of processed carbohydrates, breakfast cereals feed pathogenic bacteria and fungi in the gut, allowing them to produce their toxins.
- What about fibre? The manufacturers claim that with a bowl of their product you will get all the fibre you need. Unfortunately, it is the wrong kind of fibre for the majority of people. Fibre in breakfast cereals is full of phytates – substances that bind essential minerals and take them out of the system, thus contributing to your mineral deficiencies, which can lead to osteoporosis and other problems.[27] On top of that, fibre from grains contains lectins, substances that can damage your digestive system and the rest of the body.[28,29,30]
- There has been an interesting experiment performed in one of the food laboratories. They analysed the nutritional value of some brands of breakfast cereals and the paper boxes in which these cereals were packaged. The analysis showed that the box, made of wood pulp, had more useful nutrients in it than the cereal inside.[31] Indeed, breakfast cereals have got very low nutritional value. To compensate for that the manufacturers fortify them with synthetic forms of vitamins, claiming that by eating your morning bowl of this cereal you will get all your daily requirements of those vitamins. Well, the human body is not that simple; it has been designed to recognise and use natural vitamins that arrive in natural food form. That is why synthetic vitamins have a very low absorption rate, which means that most of them go through and out of your digestive tract without doing you any good.[32] Whatever vitamins do get absorbed the body often does not recognise as food, so they get taken straight to the kidneys and excreted in urine. We have a new syndrome in our modern pill-popping society – a syndrome of "expensive urine".

So, no matter what the advertisements say, there is nothing healthy in breakfast cereals for any of us.

Crisps, chips and other starchy snacks

Crisps, chips and popcorn, the backbone of children's diet nowadays, are highly processed carbohydrates with a detrimental effect on the gut flora. But that is not all: they are soaked with vegetable oil that has been heated to a very high temperature. Any plant oil that has been heated contains substances called trans fatty acids, which are unsaturated fatty acids with an altered chemical structure. We have talked about trans fats in previous chapters. They replace the vital omega-3 and omega-6 fatty acids in the cellular structure, making the cells dysfunctional. Consuming trans fatty acids has a direct damaging effect on the immune system. Cancer, heart disease, eczema, asthma and many neurological and psychiatric conditions have been linked to trans fats in the diet.[33]

Recently, another strong argument appeared against consuming crisps, chips and other processed carbohydrates – the acrylamides.

The acrylamides story

In the spring of 2002 the Swedish National Food Administration and Stockholm University reported that they had found highly neurotoxic and carcinogenic substances in potato crisps, French fries, bread and other baked and fried starchy foods. These substances are acrylamides.[34,35] Scientists in Norway, UK and Switzerland have confirmed this finding. They have also found acrylamides in breakfast cereals and other starchy foods that have been fried or baked at high temperatures. Recently, instant coffee has been added to the list of foods containing these highly dangerous substances. The World Health Organisation, United Nations Food and Agriculture Organisation and the US Food and Drug Administration have developed a plan to identify how acrylamides are formed in foods and what can be done to eliminate them, since they can cause cancer, neurological damage and infertility. Acrylamides are so harmful to health that there are certain maximum limits set for these substances in food packaging materials.[34,35] For years government agencies paid a lot of attention to controlling the amount of acrylamides in plastic food packaging, but nobody looked at the food inside that packaging. Now it has been discovered that some foods inside these plastic packets have incredibly high amounts of acrylamides – way above all allowed limits.[35,36] The acrylamides story provides another reason for us to avoid crisps, chips and other starchy snack foods.

Wheat

Virtually nobody buys wheat as a grain and cooks it at home; we buy foods made out of wheat flour. Wheat flour is the main ingredient in most processed carbohydrates. The flour arrives at bakeries in pre-packaged mixes for different kinds of breads, biscuits and pastries. These mixtures are already processed, with the best nutrients lost. Then they are "enriched" with preservatives, pesticides to keep insects away, chemical substances to prevent it absorbing moisture, colour and flavour improvers and softeners, just to mention a few. The bakery makes breads, pastries, cakes, biscuits, etc., from these chemical cocktails for us to eat, adding more processed ingredients on the way. Wheat flour digests and absorbs very quickly and will overload your system with glucose. For example, a slice of a typical white bread will give you the equivalent of about 5 teaspoons of sugar, which goes quickly into your bloodstream, leading to hyperinsulinemia and metabolic syndrome.[37] Wheat flour is present in most processed foods. It has become so pervasive in Western culture, that the majority of us don't realise just how much of it we consume on a daily basis. We eat wheat cereal and toast for breakfast, sandwiches and baguettes for lunch, pasta for dinner and biscuits and cakes in between: about 70 to 85% of everything entering many people's mouths daily is wheat.[31] Our physiology has not been designed to consume so much of one particular substance at the expense of everything else! People know that they should consume more fruit and vegetables, but the problem is that their stomachs are filled with wheat all day long and there is no room left for fruit and vegetables. As almost 100% of wheat products are highly processed foods, it is wheat that makes up the bulk of our health-damaging processed diets today. There is no doubt that foods made from wheat flour are a major contributor to the metabolic syndrome and atherosclerosis, as well as to every other degenerative disease on this planet.[31,32]

Sugar and anything made with it

Sugar was once called a "white death".[37] It deserves 100% of this title. The world consumption of sugar has grown to enormous proportions in the last century – 171 million metric tonnes.[38] Sugar is everywhere, and it is hard to find any processed food without it. Apart from overloading the body with glucose, causing the blood glucose roller-coaster and having a detrimental effect on the gut flora, it has been shown to have a directly damaging effect on the immune system.[24,37] On top of that, to deal with the sugar onslaught, the body has to use available minerals, vitamins and enzymes at an alarming rate, finishing up by being depleted of these vital substances.

Let us see how that happens.

In order to metabolise only one molecule of sugar, your body requires around 56 molecules of magnesium, dozens of molecules of vitamins, enzymes, minerals and other nutrients.[24,32,37,39] When we analyse a piece of fresh sugar cane or sugar beet in their natural state in a laboratory, we find that every molecule of sugar in them is indeed equipped with 56 molecules of magnesium and all those other nutrients.[40,41] So, when we eat natural sugar cane and sugar beet without processing them, the sugar in these plants gets used by the body well and brings us only health. But we do not eat sugar beet or sugar cane in their natural form. We extract the sugar out of them and throw everything else away. That pure sugar comes into the body like a villain, like a highway robber pulling nutrients out of our bones, muscles, brain and other tissues in order to be metabolised.[24,32] It needs those 56 molecules of magnesium! Where is all that magnesium going to come from? From your bones, your muscles and other organs. Consumption of sugar is a major reason for the widespread magnesium deficiency in our modern society, leading to high blood pressure, heart attacks, strokes, neurological, immune and many other problems, discussed in the previous chapter.[42,43] And this is only magnesium we have discussed. What about all the other nutrients which will be depleted in your body as a result of eating sugar? Their deficiencies will bring you many other symptoms and health problems.[44]

Cakes, sweets, and other confectioneries are made with sugar and wheat flour as the main ingredients, plus lots of chemicals (colours, preservatives, flavourings, etc.). It goes without saying that they should be out of the diet if we are to prevent atherosclerosis and every other modern disease.

Soft drinks (pops, cordials, lemonades, etc.) are a major source of sugar in our modern diets, not to mention chemical additives. A can of soda can contain from 5 to 10 teaspoons of sugar.[45] Consumption of soft drinks is one of the main reasons for our epidemics of metabolic syndrome and obesity, particularly in children. When we are thirsty our bodies need water, not sugary, chemical concoctions in colourful bottles. Commercial fruit juices are no better: they are full of processed fruit sugars and moulds.[46] Unless freshly pressed, they should not be in your diet either. While we are talking about drinks, it makes sense to mention beer. Beer is made from grains and sugar and is full of partially broken-down starch. It presents your body with a double whammy of a highly processed carbohydrate in combination with alcohol. It causes metabolic syndrome in the body: the so-called "beer belly" is one of the signs of this disorder. Consumption of beer is a major factor in our obesity, diabetes and heart disease epidemics.[37,44,45] So, if you would like to avoid those disorders you have to say goodbye to beer, or make its consumption very occasional.

As people become aware of the harmful effects of sugar on health, the industry keeps coming up with various new chemical sweeteners and puts them into food production using powerful marketing tools. It usually takes science a few years to find out about their damaging effects on health. A good example is saccharine. It had been on the market for decades before science found that it causes cancer.[47] Another example is aspartame, a sugar replacement in so-called "diet" drinks. It has been found to be carcinogenic and neurotoxic; it has been particularly implicated in our epidemic of multiple sclerosis.[48,49,50,51] Another modern sweetener is high fructose corn syrup (HFCS). Despite the fact that it has been proven to cause just about every chronic disease on the planet, it continues being used extensively by the food industry in processed foods and soft drinks.[52,53] It is best to avoid all man-made sweeteners as they are not natural to our physiology. Mother Nature gave us good healthy sweeteners, which we will discuss later.

Processed fats

All margarines, butter replacements, spreadable butter, vegetable oils, cooking oils, hydrogenated oils, shortenings and many other artificial fats are processed fats, which are alien to our human physiology and must not be consumed if we want to avoid atherosclerosis, its deadly complications and every other modern degenerative disease.[54,55] You will find processed fats in most processed foods: breads and pastries, chocolates, ice cream, biscuits, cakes, pre-prepared meals, crisps, snacks, popcorn, sauces, mayonnaise, condiments, all fried foods, baby formula, vegetarian foods, etc.

The basis of all processed fats are cooking oils and vegetable oils.[56] Cooking oils and vegetable oils are extracted from plants. All plant oils contain very fragile polyunsaturated fatty acids which are easily damaged by heat, light and oxygen.[54] That is why Mother Nature has hidden them away very carefully in the cellular structure of plants; in their oily seeds, leaves, stems and roots. When we eat plants in their natural form we get these oils in their pristine state and they are very good for us. But when we take plants to our big factories and extract the oils from them, something very different happens. Very high temperatures, pressure and various chemicals are employed which change the structure of fragile fatty acids in the plant matter creating a plethora of unnatural, chemically mutilated, harmful fats.[54,56] Then these chemically mutilated oils are put into bottles and sold in super-markets as cooking oils and vegetables oils, and added to all processed foods.

From the very beginning of these oils appearing in the human food chain worried scientific studies started coming out demonstrating that industrial vegetable oils cause cancer, heart disease, diabetes, neuro-logical damage, immune abnormalities and other health prob-lems.[57,58,59,60,61] These oils are full of chemically changed fatty acids which our human bodies are not meant to have!

Many of these changed fats in vegetable oils have not even been studied yet and we don't know what havoc they can wreak in the body. However, a group, called trans fats, has received a great deal of attention.[62,63,64] These are unsaturated fatty acids whose chemical structure has been changed through processing. Trans fatty acids are very similar in their structure to their natural counterparts, but they are somewhat "back to front". Because of their similarity they occupy the place of essential fats in the body, while being unable to do their jobs. That, in a way, makes cells disabled.[54] All organs and tissues in the body are affected. For example, trans fats have great immune-suppressing ability, playing a detrimental role in many different functions of the immune system.[62] They have been implicated in diabetes, atherosclerosis, cancer and neurological and psychiatric conditions.[62,66] They interfere with pregnancy and conception, the normal production of hormones, the ability of insulin to respond to glucose and the ability of enzymes and other active substances to do their jobs.[62] They have damaging effects on the liver and kidneys.[62] A breast-feeding mother would have trans fats in her milk fairly soon after ingesting a helping of a "healthy" butter replacement.[54,62] A baby's brain has a very high percentage of unsaturated fatty acids; trans fats would replace them and interfere with the brain development. There is simply no safe limit of trans fats in the diet. And yet a packet of crisps will provide you with about 6 grams of trans fats, a small snack packet of cookies will give you 7–12 grams, a snack packet of processed cheese (mainly advertised to children) will provide 8 grams of trans fats, a tablespoon of a common margarine will give you 4–6 grams, a portion of French fries, cooked in vegetable oil will serve you with 8–9 grams of trans fats.[54,64] Given their ability to impair bodily functions on the most basic biochemical levels, there is no doubt that their role in our modern epidemics of degenerative disease is greatly underestimated. Trans fats and other processed fats will directly cause endothelial injury in your body and atherosclerosis.[65,66]

In order to make vegetable and cooking oils look solid and prolong their shelf life, they are hydrogenated.[63] Hydrogenation is a process of adding hydrogen molecules to the chemical structure of oils under high pressure at a very high temperature – 120–210^{0}C (248–410^{0}F) – in the presence of nickel, aluminium and sometimes other metals. Remnants of these toxic metals stay in the hydrogenated oils, adding to the general toxic load, which the body then has to work hard to get rid of.[54] Hydrogenation of vegetable oils creates products which are even more toxic and harmful to health.

Consumption of large amounts of vegetable and cooking oils presents another problem for the body: the excess of omega-6 fatty acids.[55,67] To be healthy our bodies require a very delicate balance between different fatty acids. When we eat plants in their natural state the oils we consume from them do not upset that balance. But when we eat processed foods full of vegetable cooking oils we receive excessive amounts of omega-6 fats, which contribute to a pro-inflammatory environment in the body and lead to disease.[54,55,67]

In the following chapters we will talk about what fats are good for us, humans, to consume.

Processed salt

Only a small percentage of all industrial salt production goes for human consumption. More than 90% of all salt produced is used for industrial applications: the making of soaps, detergents, plastics, agricultural chemicals, PVC, etc., etc.[82] These industrial applications require pure sodium chloride. However, salt in Nature contains many other elements: in fact natural crystal salt and whole sea salt contain all the minerals and trace elements which the human body is made of.[84,85] In this natural state salt is not only good for us, but essential. Because the industry requires pure sodium chloride, all the other elements and minerals get removed from the natural salt. We consume it under the name of "table salt" and of course all our processed foods contain plenty of it.[84]

This kind of salt comes into the body like a villain upsetting our homeostasis on the most basic level.[88,91] Our bodies have been designed to receive sodium chloride in combination with all the other minerals and trace elements that a natural salt would provide.[83,84,85] Pure sodium chloride draws water to itself and causes water retention with many consequences, such as high blood pressure, tissue oedema and poor circulation.[87,89] As the body tries to deal with the excess of sodium chloride, various harmful acids and gall bladder and kidney stones are formed.[86,87] As sodium in the body works in a team with many other minerals and trace elements (potassium, calcium, magnesium, copper, zinc, manganese, etc.), the levels of those substances get out of normal balance.[84,87,90] The harmful results of table salt consumption can be numerous and very serious. That is why most medical practitioners, including the mainstream doctors, tell us not to consume table salt.

Our planet has plenty of good quality salt for us to consume. Throughout human history, salt was highly valued: it used to be called "the white gold", the Roman Empire paid its soldiers with salt (hence the word "salary").[83,85] Natural salt is just as fundamental to our physiology as water is.[92,93] We need to consume salt in its natural state: as a crystal salt from salt mines or as a whole unprocessed sea salt. There are number of companies around the world that can provide you with good quality natural salt.

No soya, please!

Soya is very big business, particularly in the USA. A large percentage of the industry uses genetically modified soya.[68] Soya is cheap to produce and, following some research showing that it can be beneficial for menopausal women, the whole market has exploded with soya products. Soya can be found in many processed foods, margarines, salad dressings and sauces, breads, biscuits, pizza, baby food, children's snacks, sweets, cakes, vegetarian products, dairy replacements, infant milk formulas, etc. Is there a problem with that? Let us have a look at some facts.

1. In Japan and other eastern cultures soya is traditionally used as a whole bean or fermented as soy sauce, tofu, natto, miso and tempeh.[69] The form in which soya is used in the West is called *soy protein isolate*.[70] How is it made? After removing the fibre with an alkaline solution, the soya beans are put into large aluminium tanks with an acid wash. Acid makes the soy beans absorb aluminium, which will remain in the end product.[68] Aluminium has been linked to dementia and Alzheimer's disease, and indeed there has been a lot of publicity recently that links soya consumption with these mental disorders.[71,72] After the aluminium-acid wash the beans are treated with many other chemicals, including nitrates, which have been implicated in cancer development. The end product is an almost tasteless powder, easy to use and add to any food.

The majority of processed foods contain this powder, and of course soya milk, yogurt and soya infant formulas are made out of it.[68] It is a highly processed substance with poor nutritional value and a lot of harmful qualities. Animals fed this product die from cancer and malnourishment and produce sick offspring.[68,73] Recently its consumption has been linked to cancer, inflammation and other degenerative conditions in humans.[68,73,74,75]

2. Soya is a natural goitrogen. What does it mean? It means that soya has an ability to impair thyroid function. Low thyroid function has very serious implications for your health, including the development of atherosclerosis.[68,73,75,76]

3. Soya beans have a very high concentration of phytates. These substances are found in all grains as well, particularly in their bran. Phytates have a great ability to bind to minerals, which prevents them from being absorbed, particularly calcium, magnesium, iron and zinc.[68,77,78]

4. Soya has gained its popularity as a treatment for menopause because it contains plant oestrogens, which do not work in the body in the same way as their natural counterparts do. It is questionable whether these substances are indeed useful for menopausal women. For the rest of us, particularly for men and children, they are most definitely harmful. There is a growing concern among health professionals about the quantity of plant oestogens infants and small children might be getting from soya milk and infant formulas.[76,79,80]

5. Western producers of soy would like you to believe that the health of Japanese people depends on their consumption of soya. The truth is very different. Soya is consumed largely in a fermented form and in small amounts. Many of the health benefits of traditional Japanese cooking can be attributed to seafood and seaweed, which is consumed daily in good amounts. Fresh and dried seaweed is full of nutrients and is extensively used in cooking in Japan and many other cultures of the world.[81]

If you want to eat soya, have it only in the natural, traditional fermented form as soy sauce, natto, miso, tofu and tempeh. These foods are prepared according to traditional wisdom, which has served people in the East for centuries.

What should we eat to prevent atherosclerosis and its deadly complications?

Let's start with shopping. Buy your food in the shape and form that Nature has made it and prepare it yourself at home, using traditional methods of cooking: on the stove, the grill or in the oven. Avoid microwaves as they destroy food and can make it carcinogenic.[1,2]
What should we buy?

1. Buy meats, fresh or frozen, including game and organ meats

Avoid all mainstream processed meats: hams, bacons, sausages, delicatessen, tinned meats, etc. because they are full of preservatives and other chemicals that have been proven to cause endothelial dysfunction, cancer and other problems.[4,5] Meats prepared in a traditional way using natural salt and fermentation are safe to eat and taste much better. Avoid genetically modified meats. Our physiology has been designed to have meats as Nature designed them – without antibiotics, pesticides and other chemicals. Look for natural grass-fed meats, preferably organic. Avoid lean meats; our physiology can only use meat fibres when they come with the fat, collagen and other substances that a proper piece of meat will provide.[3] When we eat poultry it is important to eat the skin and the fats, as well as the meat; and the most valuable nutrients come from the legs, wings, skin and carcase of the bird, not so much from the breast.[6] If you want sausages, find a local butcher who will make them for you on order with just minced meat (full fat), salt, pepper, chopped onion and any fresh herbs of your choice. Order them in bulk and keep them in the freezer. Once you have tasted these sausages you will never want to eat the commercial ones again (full of wheat and chemicals). Contrary to popular belief, it is meats, fish and other animal products that have the highest content of vitamins, amino acids, nourishing fats, many minerals and other nutrients which we humans need on a daily basis.[3] All this nutrition in meats and fish also comes in the most digestible form for us humans. I find it deceptive when vitamin tables in some books on nutrition show that plant foods (grains, vegetables, fruit, etc.) provide all our vitamins. First of all, the form in which plants contain these vitamins is difficult for us to digest. Secondly, if you compare the amounts of vitamins in meat, fish or other animal products with plant foods, it is the animal products that are at the top of the list. Let us have a look at just some of them. [3,7]

Vitamin B1 (thiamin): the richest sources are pork, liver, heart and kidneys.
Vitamin B2 (riboflavin): the richest sources are eggs, meat, milk, poultry and fish.
Vitamin B3 (niacin): the richest sources are meat and poultry.
Vitamin B5 (pantothenic acid): the richest sources are meats and liver.
Vitamin B6 (pyridoxine): the richest sources are meat, poultry, fish and eggs.
Vitamin B12 (cyanocobalamin): the richest sources are meat, poultry, fish, eggs and milk.
Biotin: the richest sources are liver and egg yolks.
Vitamin A: the richest sources are liver, fish, egg yolks and butter. We are talking about the real vitamin A, which is ready for the body to use. You will see in many publications that you can get your vitamin A from fruit and vegetables in the form of carotenoids. The problem is that carotenoids have to be converted into real vitamin A in the body, and a lot of us are unable to do this conversion, because we are too toxic, or because we have an ongoing inflammation in the body. [8] So, if you do not consume animal products with the real vitamin A, then you may develop a deficiency in this vital vitamin despite eating lots of carrots. Vitamin A deficiency will lead to impaired immunity and development of atherosclerosis. [7,8,9]
Vitamin D: the richest food sources are fish liver oils, eggs and fish.
Vitamin K2 (menaquinone): the richest sources are organ meats, full fat cheese, good quality butter and cream (yellow from grass-fed animals), animal fats and egg yolks. This vitamin is essential for heart health, its deficiency leads to deposition of calcium in the arteries and initiation of inflammation.[10] Apart from the high fat foods an important source of this vitamin is our own gut flora: the probiotic bacteria in the gut produce and release vitamin K2. Fermented foods are full of vitamin K2 as the bacteria produce it in the process of fermentation; natto (fermented soy beans) is one of the richest sources in the Eastern

culture while in the West well-aged natural full-fat cheese is a good source of this vitamin. [9,10]

All these vitamins are absolutely essential for us, humans; we cannot live without them, let alone function well. Three well-researched vitamins, which are generally thought to come from plants, are vitamin C, folate and vitamin K1 (phylloquinone). However, now we know that liver contains high amounts of both vitamin C and folate.[7,9] Sweet fruit generally interfere with the digestion of meats and should be eaten between meals. Vegetables, however, combine with meats and fish very well and will provide the missing nutrients. There is another important reason for eating meats and fish with vegetables, which is the way we metabolise food. After digesting and utilising meats and fish, our body tissues accumulate acids. After digesting most vegetables, our body becomes alkaline. By combining the meats and vegetables in one meal we balance the acidity in the body, which is important because both too acid and too alkaline states are not very healthy.[9,11] Raw vegetables have stronger alkalising ability than cooked ones.

Fresh liver is an absolute powerhouse of nutrition for our physiology and should be consumed on a regular basis, particularly by people with nutritional deficiencies. People with anaemia should have fresh liver and red meats daily (lamb, beef, game and organ meats in particular) because these foods are the best remedy for anaemia.[3,8] They not only provide iron in the haem form, the form which the human body absorbs best, but they also provide the B vitamins and other nutrients essential for treating anaemia. Meats also promote better absorption of non-haem iron from vegetables and fruit, while vitamin C from vegetables and greens promotes absorption of iron from meats.[3,9] Large epidemiological studies show that eating red meat is associated with a much lower incidence of iron deficiency and anaemia in various countries of the world.[3]

The misinformation about meats, particularly red meats, has been driven by commercial powers, who profit from replacing these natural foods with their processed alternatives. Fresh, natural meats have nothing to do with heart disease, atherosclerosis, cancer or any other disease, and are important for us to eat in order to provide all the nutrients we humans need.[12,13]

Home-made meat stock is a wonderful nutritional and digestive remedy, something our grandmothers used to make on a daily basis. The best stock is made from bones, joints and offcuts. All you have to do is boil them on a low heat for 2–3 hours in plenty of water, with some added salt and pepper. As you cook bones, joints and meats in water, the nutrients from them get extracted into the water. The resulting stock is rich in collagen, gelatine, minerals, amino acids and many other nutrients, which have a healing effect on your digestive system, your joints, your brain, your immunity and your endothelium.[12,14] Use these meat stocks for making soups, stews and simply as a warming therapeutic drink with and between meals. Chicken stock made from a whole chicken is the best remedy for any cold or tummy upset. It goes without saying that all commercially available stock granules and cubes are to be avoided. They do not possess any of the healing properties of a home-made meat stock and are full of detrimental ingredients. Meats cooked in water are easier to digest for a person with a sensitive digestive system.[15]

2. Buy fish and shellfish fresh or frozen

Avoid tinned, cooked, dyed and other processed fish and shellfish. Wild fish is always better than farmed. There is a question, however, about the mercury and other pollutants that we pump into our oceans and rivers. For that reason some official bodies recommend limiting fish consumption.[16] However, research shows that people who consume more fish are in better health than people who limit it.[17] A healthy human body has a good ability to handle pollutants and remove them. The first and the best barrier to any pollution coming with food is healthy gut flora.[18] The beneficial bacteria in our gut flora have an excellent ability to bind, neutralise and remove from the body mercury, lead and other heavy metals and toxins. However, in people with damaged gut flora these poisons remain in the body, so restoring normal gut flora is very important, particularly after a course of antibiotics.[19] To limit your exposure to environmental toxins it makes sense to avoid large carnivorous fish, such as tuna, shark and swordfish, as they accumulate far more pollutants than small fish.[20,21] Smaller fish, such as oily fish (sardines, mackerel and herring) and any other wild fish, are important for us to eat on a regular basis. They provide us with good proteins, minerals and essential fats. Fish oils are the best anti-inflammatory remedies Nature has given us and they work best when consumed as part of the whole fish.[22,23]

3. Buy fresh eggs from free-range hens, preferably organic

Eggs are a wonder food, full of easy-to-digest nutrition. A fresh, raw egg yolk has been compared with human breast milk: it is absorbed literally without needing digestion and provides you with almost every nutrient under the sun in the best possible biochemical form.[24] As already mentioned, raw eggs have traditionally been used as a cure for tuberculosis because they provide powerful immune-boosting nutrients.[26] Any person with memory loss must have at least three, preferably five to six fresh eggs a day. It has been demonstrated in a number of clinical trials that eating fresh eggs improves memory.[25] Learning ability and behaviour in children can be improved tremendously by consumption of fresh eggs.[28] Children should have at least two eggs a day. The faulty diet-heart hypothesis has scared people away from eating eggs because they contain cholesterol. We have already discussed the subject of cholesterol. The story that it "causes" heart disease is an absolute fallacy; cholesterol is an essential-to-life substance, and eating dietary cholesterol is no more harmful than drinking water.[27] It goes without saying that you must avoid any processed eggs: dried egg powders, mixes, etc. Fresh eggs are an excellent food for breakfast, cooked any way you like. Served with a fresh salad and plenty of cold-pressed virgin olive oil, eggs will set your blood sugar and body biochemistry at a normal level for the day.

4. Buy fresh vegetables, not frozen, tinned, cooked or otherwise processed

French artichoke, beets, asparagus, broccoli, Brussels sprouts, cabbage, cauliflower, carrots, cucumber, celery, marrow, courgette (zucchini), aubergine (eggplant), garlic, onions, kale, lettuce, mushrooms, parsley, green peas, peppers of all colours, pumpkin, squash, spinach, tomatoes, turnips, watercress and other low-starch vegetables are your best choices.

There is a mountain of information available on the benefits of eating vegetables, as they contain a plethora of wonderful nutrients.[24,28] They should be eaten every day, both cooked and raw. Cooked vegetables are easier to digest and provide warm nourishment for the body, while raw vegetables keep our bodies clean inside as they provide powerful detoxifying substances and the best quality fibre.[28] In cold weather and when you have a cold, eat plenty of warming soups and stews with well-cooked vegetables. Cold salads do not agree with our physiology in those conditions. However, in hot weather cold salads are exactly what we need. The best vegetables come from people's private gardens: fresh, in season and usually organic. Vegetables that have to travel half across the world to reach your table are not in the same league in any possible way.

Try to replace wheat products, such as bread, pasta, pastries, pies, biscuits, etc., with vegetables and your body will reward you in a matter of days with better health, more energy, clearer thinking and good sleep.[24,25,28]

5. Buy fresh fruit, not cooked, tinned, frozen or processed in any way

Fruit needs to be ripe! Unripe fruit is difficult to digest. You have to understand that anything you cannot digest properly will do you no good. Unfortunately a lot of fruit in your supermarket is likely to be unripe.

Sweet and tropical fruits should be consumed between meals as they may interfere with the digestion of meats.[25] The exceptions are avocado, tomato, lemon and other fruits that do not taste sweet. People who have abnormal gut flora often cannot digest different fruits, and have to avoid them. Once you take steps to improve your gut flora, you may be able to eat fruits that you could not tolerate before (we will talk about gut flora in the following chapters). Just like vegetables, the best fruit comes from people's private gardens – fresh, organic, picked ripe and full of nutrients. Commercially produced fruit is likely to be sprayed with chemicals, picked unripe and grown on exhausted soils. That is why commercial fruit is difficult to digest and is a poor source of nutrition.

Organic is always better than non-organic. I know a lot of people who could not tolerate various fruit and vegetables until they switched to their organic counterparts.

Berries are a wonderful variety of fruit, absolutely packed with essential nutrients.[24,25] Raspberries, black, red and white currants, gooseberries, elderberries, blackberries, strawberries, etc. are full of vitamins, antioxidants, minerals and many other substances that will regulate your blood sugar level and keep your body clean on the inside. Regular consumption of *uncooked* fresh or frozen berries will prevent endothelial dysfunction, atherosclerosis, cancer and many other maladies.[28,29] Take any chance to pick your own berries in season and freeze them for the winter. When you want to have jam, just defrost some berries and mix them with honey to taste. Make just enough to consume in a few days because this jam will not keep for long.

6. Buy natural organic dairy

Unprocessed milk, unprocessed cream, fresh natural butter (not spreadable and not butter substitutes), natural ghee, natural live yoghurt, kefir and natural cheeses produced in a traditional way. Avoid all processed cheeses, dried and long-life milk and cream, and other long-life or processed dairy.

One processing that most commercial milk is subjected to nowadays is homogenisation, when the milk is forced through a fine mesh to break down the fat globules. This is done purely for cosmetic purposes and removes the milk one more step away from its natural state, making it more processed.[32,33] It is particularly important to stick to organic dairy, as milk accumulates most chemicals that non-organic cows are exposed to.[31]

Dairy products are full of wonderful nutrition and are important for us to eat.[24] However, a lot of people cannot tolerate milk. This is because commonly available milk has been pasteurised. Pasteurisation destroys milk: it changes the chemical structure of its proteins, fats and carbohydrates, kills beneficial bacteria and destroys enzymes and vitamins.[30,36] Pasteurised milk is difficult for most of us to digest, particularly infants and children. That is why milk allergy and intolerance is so common. Unprocessed, unpasteurised, straight-from-the-cow milk is very easy to digest as it contains enzymes that digest the milk for you to some degree.[34,35] However, this milk must be organic! Non-organic cows often have mastitis, so a lot of pus and infectious organisms finish up in their milk. This kind of milk has to be pasteurised.[31] Organic grass-fed cows are healthy and their milk is free from infections; it does not need pasteurisation. There is a growing number of farmers around the world who produce organic, unprocessed, unpasteurised milk from grass-fed cows.[31,61] If you look for such a farmer in your area you may be surprised to find one without too much difficulty.

Milk contains a sugar, called lactose. Some people get diagnosed as lactose intolerant. Well, after the infancy we are all "lactose intolerant" because the human gut does not produce an enzyme to digest lactose, called lactase.[37] So, how do many of us manage to digest milk? Because we have particular species of probiotic bacteria in the gut, which do this work for us. Some of the most well-studied lactose-digesting species are physiological strains of E. coli.[38] People, who cannot digest lactose have abnormal gut flora, they are lacking those probiotic bacteria. Instead of sentencing yourself to consuming highly processed lactose-free dairy products, you need to restore your gut flora by eating fermented foods and consuming good quality probiotics (read more on this subject in the next chapter). Fermented dairy products, such as live yoghurt, kefir, natural traditional cheeses and butter have greatly reduced lactose contents and are usually tolerated well by lactose-intolerant people.[39] Pasteurisation of milk is a major contributor to lactose intolerance in the population. Raw fresh milk contains an active enzyme lactase to digest the lactose for you, but this enzyme is destroyed by pasteurisation. Many lactose-intolerant people find that they can digest raw milk perfectly well, while pasteurised milk causes all the usual unpleasant symptoms of lactose intolerance (bloating, indigestion, abdominal pain and diarrhoea).[34,36,37]

7. Buy unprocessed nuts and oily seeds

Walnuts, almonds, brazil nuts, pecans, hazelnuts, cashew nuts, chestnuts, peanuts, sunflower seeds, pumpkin seeds, sesame seeds, etc. Do not buy them cooked, roasted, salted, coated or processed in any other way; buy them just shelled or in their shells. Nuts, sunflower, sesame and pumpkin seeds can be ground into flour consistency and used for making breads and cakes at home (please, look in the recipe section). Nuts and seeds are full of vital nutrients and are very important for us to eat. There is a mountain of research to show that regular consumption of these foods prevents heart disease, atherosclerosis, cancer, auto-immune disorders and many other health problems.[40,41,42,43]

It is not difficult to make nuts a normal part of your diet: just put a mixture of nuts, seeds and dried fruit into an attractive bowl and keep it on your coffee table in front of the TV set. You will be surprised how quickly your family gets used to snacking on these health-giving foods, instead of eating harmful, commercial processed snacks.

Keep in mind that nuts and seeds are very fibrous and can be difficult to digest. If you have digestive problems please study the GAPS Diet in my book *Gut And Psychology Syndrome*.[44]

8. Buy organic beans and pulses

Buy them in their whole natural form and cook them at home. Avoid commercially available tinned beans and pulses, as they are processed foods full of sugar and other additives. Before cooking, all beans and pulses have to be pre-soaked in water for at least 12 hours to reduce amounts of lectins and other harmful substances.[45,46] After soaking, rinse well under running water. Once cooked, they can be used in many recipes including baking bread and cakes. Avoid commercial flours made out of beans and pulses, as they have not been pre-soaked before grinding. There are many wonderful traditional recipes for cooking beans and pulses. However, if you have digestive problems, you may find them difficult to digest. For this reason many of the world's traditional cultures ferment their beans and pulses, which makes them easy to digest, even for babies.[45]

9. Buy and use only natural fats

We are talking about the fats that Mother Nature provided, and which traditional cultures around the world have been using for millennia: animal fats, fats on meats, butter and ghee, coconut and palm oil, *cold-pressed virgin* olive oil and other *cold-pressed virgin* natural oils (flax, hemp, avocado, evening primrose, walnut, sunflower, etc.).

Cold-pressed oils are difficult to produce and, therefore, are expensive. They are full of very fragile health-giving substances and must not be used for cooking as heat would destroy them. They are also easily damaged by oxygen and light, so we have to extract them with minimum exposure to air and keep them refrigerated in dark glass bottles.[47] Use these cold-pressed oils in small amounts as a dressing on ready served meals or take them as a supplement. They will provide you with essential fatty acids, antioxidants and many other good things. However, the majority of us don't have to buy these oils at all. Just eating fresh nuts, seeds (particularly sprouted), green leafy vegetables and other fresh vegetables, berries and other fresh fruit will provide you with **essential fatty acids**: alpha-linolenic acid (omega-3) and linoleic acid (omega-6). We cannot live without them and our bodies cannot produce them (as far as we know at the moment), so we must get them from food. That is why they are called essential.[47] In a healthy body these parent oils get converted to their derivatives, which the body also cannot live without. The problem is that many of us cannot do this conversion because we fill our bodies with man-made toxins, making this process impossible; at the same time, due to our modern diet, we have deficiencies in vitamins, minerals and other nutrients required for the conversion.[48] That is why we have to eat those derivatives in a ready-made form, which is why they are called **conditionally essential fatty acids**. These are: EPA (eicosapentaenoic acid, omega-3), DHA (docosahexaenoic acid, omega-3), GLA (gamma-linolenic acid, omega-6) and AA (arachidonic acid, omega-6). People with any inflammatory problem in the body, such as atherosclerosis and heart disease; any immune problem, such as arthritis, asthma and allergies; any neurological and psychiatric condition; and any other chronic degenerative disease typically cannot do the conversion. That is why they must consume these conditionally essential fatty acids, as well as the parent ones, on a daily basis.[49]

EPA and DHA come from fresh fish, particularly oily fish, and there are many good quality fish oil supplements on the market.

GLA comes from seeds and nuts, particularly rich sources are borage oil (24%), blackcurrant seed oil (18%), evening primrose oil (9%) and hemp oil (2%).[47]

AA comes from animal products: butter, cream, eggs and fats on meats. AA makes about 12% of the brain fat and is essential for us to consume daily, particularly for people with memory problems and any neurological and psychiatric condition.[50] AA is an important part of our immune system, as well as many other organs and systems in the body.[51] Unfortunately, there is a lot of misinformation about AA because it comes from animal fats. Some popular health writers recommend avoiding AA by throwing away the egg yolks and eating only the egg whites, as well as avoiding all dairy and animal fats. This propaganda is not based on any real science and does not make any sense: if AA was bad for us, then why did Mother Nature put it into so many foods that we humans have thrived on for millennia? There is a simplistic idea that AA creates so-called "bad eicosanoids" in the body. The science on eicosanoids is very young and by no means complete yet; it is very unwise to rely on it, let alone make any changes in your lifestyle based on it.[52] In my clinical experience I see in **all** of my patients that adding plenty of natural foods rich in AA is essential for their recovery.

Avoid all vegetable and cooking oils, widely available in supermarkets. They are extremely processed substances full of trans fats, solvents and other harmful chemicals. Consumption of these oils and margarines is one of the main causes of our heart disease epidemic.[53,54,55,56,57,58]

So, what fats do we use for cooking?

Cook with animal fats, such as lard, pork dripping, lamb fat, beef fat, goose fat, duck fat, etc. It is best to do what our grandmothers did: collect the fats yourself after cooking your meats; they will keep in a glass jar in your refrigerator for a long time and are excellent to use for cooking. Roasting a duck will provide you with a cup of excellent fat, which has been proven to be heart protective.[47,59] Roasting a large goose will provide you with almost half a year's supply of an excellent cooking fat. You can buy some of these fats from a traditional butcher. You can also cook with butter, ghee, natural coconut oil and palm oil. All these fats are healthy for us and very stable: they generally do not change their chemical structure when we cook with them, they can even be reused.[47]

I almost hear you asking a number of very common questions: "What about the 'deadly' saturated fats? Don't they cause heart disease? Aren't animal fats all saturated?"

This is the result of the relentless efforts made by the food industry to fight their competition. What is their competition? The natural fats, of course. There is not much profit to be made from the natural fats, while processed oils and fats bring very good profits.[53] So, it is in the food industry's interest to convince everybody that natural fats are harmful for health, while their processed fats, hydrogenated and cooking oils are good for us.[55] We have been subjected to this propaganda for almost a century now; no wonder that many of us have succumbed to it.

The saturated fats in particular were singled out by the food industry. How did that happen? The late Dr Mary Enig, an international expert in lipid biochemistry, explained: "In the late 1950s, an American researcher, Ancel Keys, announced that the CHD epidemic was being caused by the hydrogenated vegetable fats; previously this same person had introduced the idea that saturated fat was the culprit. The edible oil industry quickly responded to this perceived threat to their products by mounting a public relations campaign to promote the belief that it was only the saturated fatty acid component in the hydrogenated oils that was causing the problem... From that time on, the edible fats and oils industry promoted the twin ideas that saturates (namely animal and dairy fats) were troublesome, and polyunsaturates (mainly corn oil and later soybean oil) were health-giving".[47]

The wealthy food giants spend billions on employing an army of "scientists" to provide them with "scientific proof" of their claims. In the meantime the real science was, and is, providing us with the truth. However, it is the food giants who have the money to advertise their "science" in all the popular media. Real science is too poor to spend money on that. As a result, the population hears only what the commercial powers want them to hear.

So, what is the truth? What does real science tell us?

1. Processed fats, hydrogenated fats and cooking vegetable oils cause atherosclerosis, heart disease and cancer.[55] This is a fact, proven overwhelmingly by real, honest science. All animal experiments to "prove" the diet-heart hypothesis were made with processed fats and processed oxidised cholesterol, which makes them completely invalid.[47,59]

2. Animal fats have nothing to do with heart disease, atherosclerosis and cancer. Our human physiology needs these fats; they are important for us to eat on a daily basis.[59]
3. Saturated fats are heart protective: they lower the Lp(a) in the blood, reduce calcium deposition in the arteries and are the preferred source of energy for the heart muscle.[47] Saturated fats enhance our immune system, protect us from infections and are essential for the body to be able to utilise the unsaturated omega-3 and omega-6 fatty acids.[47,59] One of the most saturated fats that Nature has provided is coconut oil. It has been shown to be wonderfully healthy and therapeutic in most degenerative conditions.[47]
4. Animal fats contain a variety of different fatty acids, not just saturated ones.[60] Pork fat is 45% monounsaturated, 11% polyunsaturated and 44% saturated. Lamb fat is 38% monounsaturated, 2% polyunsaturated and 58% saturated. Beef fat is 47% monounsaturated, 4% polyunsaturated and 49% saturated. Butter is 30% monounsaturated, 4% polyunsaturated and 52% saturated. This is the natural composition of animal fats and our bodies use every bit, including the saturated part. If you want to understand how important every bit of the animal fat is for us, let us have a look at the composition of human breast milk. The fat portion of the breast milk is 48% saturated, 33% monounsaturated and 16% polyunsaturated.[47,60] Our babies thrive beautifully on this composition of fats, and the largest part of it is saturated.
5. We need all of the natural fats in natural foods, and saturated and monounsaturated fats need to be the largest part of our fat intake.
6. The simplistic idea that eating fat makes you fat is completely wrong. Consuming processed carbohydrates causes obesity.[48,49,60] Dietary fats go into the structure of your body: your brain, bones, muscles, immune system, etc. – every cell in the body is made out of fats to a large degree.[60]

These are the facts, which honest science has provided. Unfortunately, as already mentioned, most of us do not hear about the discoveries of honest science. Spreading any information in this world costs money. So, the population at large mostly gets information that serves somebody with a fat wallet. In order to get the real, true information on any subject, we have to search for it, rather than relying on the "news" and "scientific breakthroughs" unleashed on us by the popular media.

10. Buy whole, unprocessed grains and prepare them properly before consuming!

Buckwheat, millet, quinoa, oats, barley, brown rice, etc., to be cooked at home following traditional recipes. Do not buy processed grains or anything made out of flour. The most processed grains you can buy are breakfast cereals.

Whole grains should not be consumed without proper preparation, as they contain number of harmful substances. They contain lectins, which can damage the gut wall and many other tissues and organs.[61,62] They contain phytates, which impair mineral absorption and can cause serious mineral deficiencies and bone loss; regular consumption of bran in particular is linked to osteoporosis.[63] They contain hard to digest proteins and starches. Wheat, rye, oats and barley contain a protein, called gluten, which is very difficult to digest for most of us and is positively dangerous for people with any digestive problems.[64,65] The popular advice to eat whole grains is misleading, because they are generally indigestible for humans and can do a lot of harm in the body. Herbivorous animals, which thrive on plants including whole grains, have several stomachs full of bacteria, which digest the plant matter for them.[66] We humans have only one stomach which, if it is healthy, has very little bacteria in it and has not been designed to digest grains without prior preparation. Traditional cultures around the world have known this fact for millennia and have always fermented or sprouted grains prior to cooking them. Fermentation reduces the amounts of lectins and phytates, predigests gluten and starch and releases nutrients.[67] To ferment, the grains can simply be soaked in water for several days; to speed up the process you can add a few spoonfuls of live yoghurt, kefir or whey to the water. When the grain has fermented, cook it in the usual way. Another excellent way to make grains more digestible is sprouting. Sprouting is a very easy procedure: soak the grains for 12–24 hours in water, then drain and keep moist in a warm place for a few days. As grains are seeds, they will sprout small shoots. In that form they are much more nourishing and easier to digest raw or cooked.

There is a very important point to make about grains, whether whole or not. Traditionally grains were always consumed with a good amount of natural fats: butter, ghee, olive oil, coconut or palm oil, goose fat, duck fat, pork fat, etc.[68,69] There is a lot of wisdom to that: grains are a concentrated source of carbohydrates and, unless their digestion is slowed down by fats, will absorb quite quickly, raising the blood sugar level too high, with all the damaging consequences we discussed in the previous chapter. So, the last thing you want to do is eat your grains fat free. The same goes for potatoes, sweet potatoes, yams, Jerusalem artichokes, parsnips and other starchy vegetables. They are a concentrated source of carbohydrates, so their digestion needs to be slowed down by adding good amounts of natural fats.

If you need to lose weight, suffer from diabetes or have digestive problems, avoid grains and starchy vegetables altogether (and, obviously, anything made out of them). People with any digestive problems must avoid all grains and starchy vegetables until their digestion improves.[70]

What about **bread**? The majority of people find it very difficult to avoid eating bread. People generally believe that bread is good for them because humankind has consumed it for thousands of years. The problem is that what we call bread nowadays is something very different to what humans consumed even a hundred years ago. When did you last look at the ingredients list of the bread you buy? You will find that most breads on the shelves of our supermarkets and our bakeries are extremely processed products, full of dozens of chemicals, soy protein isolate, margarine, harmful vegetable oils, modified starch, hydrogenated oils, etc., etc. Bread is probably the biggest source of processed foods that the majority of us eat today.

If you want bread, make your own, following traditional time-proven bread making recipes. These are not the recipes that come with your bread-making machine! I highly recommend a wonderful recipe book by Sally Fallon, *Nourishing Traditions*, which will provide you with traditional recipes from different cultures of the world.[69] If you live in an area where your local baker makes traditional sourdough bread, then consider yourself extremely lucky.

Remember, that if you need to lose weight, suffer from diabetes or have digestive problems, avoid grains and starchy vegetables altogether and anything made out of them. Bread made out of grains (generally wheat or rye flour) will do you no favours. However, if you bake bread using nuts and oily seeds, ground into flour consistency, you will do your body a lot of good. You can buy almond flour (ground almonds) commercially or grind nuts, sunflower and pumpkin seeds into a flour consistency. You will find some bread making recipes in the recipe section.

11. What about sweet taste?

Nature has provided us with excellent sweeteners: natural, unprocessed honey and dried fruit (make sure the fruit is natural, not coated in sugar, syrup or anything else). These sweet things are full of life-giving nutrients and do not damage the body.[69,70,72] Avoid sugar and all artificial sweeteners. If you want to bake a cake, dried fruit such as dates, figs and raisins will sweeten it for you beautifully and make your cake more nutritious.

Before the introduction of sugar in the 17th century honey was the only sweetener that humans used in their diet. Starting from the end of the 17th century, sugar, being cheaper and more available, replaced honey in people's diet, beginning an era of sugar-related health problems. Honey is natural to our physiology, and far from damaging our health it has a lot of health-giving properties. Honey has been used as food and medicine for thousands of years. In Greek mythology honey was considered a "food fit for the gods". There are dozens of books written about the health-giving properties of natural honey.[72] It works as an antiseptic and provides vitamins, minerals, amino acids and many other bioactive substances.[72,73,74] Depending on the variety of flowers, from which a particular honey has been collected, different flavour and composition of nutrients and bio-active substances can be found in the honey. Traditionally honey has been used to treat digestive disorders, chest and throat infections, arthritis, anaemia, insomnia, headaches, debility and cancer.[72,73,76,77,78,79] It can be applied therapeutically to open wounds, eczema patches, skin rashes, skin and mouth ulcers and erosions.[71,72,73,74,75]

Dried fruit will provide you with all the vitamins, minerals and other beneficial substances that fruit contains, but in concentrated amounts. As a result, in every traditional culture of the world dried fruit was used as medicine for various health problems. It was specifically given to pregnant women and to couples who were trying to conceive a baby; to people with tuberculosis and other chronic infections; to people with neurological and psychological symptoms and to people recovering from severe illness.[80,81,82,83,84] Regular consumption of dried dates, raisins, figs, currants, berries, prunes, etc. will do much more for your health than the most expensive supplements in the world. Apart from that, they are the natural sweets Mother Nature gave us. So, instead of buying commercial sweets, which damage your children's health, teach them to eat dried fruit.

12. Eat fermented foods, prepared according to traditional methods

Fermentation is the use of beneficial microbes to preserve food for long periods of time. We have already mentioned natural live yoghurt, kefir and cheese – these are fermented foods. Sauerkraut (fermented cabbage) and other fermented vegetables will provide you with wonderful nutrition and beneficial bacteria. Good quality wine, natural kvass and natural beer without additives are fermented drinks and are good for us in moderate amounts.

Traditionally every culture of the world made fermented foods: people fermented dairy, grains, meats, fish, beans, pulses, vegetables and fruit because that was the only way they could preserve food for a long time.[85] Foods used to be seasonal and there were no supermarkets where one can buy anything all year round. So, for example, when your cabbages were ready you had to do something with them, or they would rot away and you would be left without cabbage for the rest of the year. So, people made sauerkraut and consumed it until the next harvest, taking in mouthfuls of beneficial probiotic bacteria, active enzymes and other wonderful substances that only a fermented food would provide.[69,85] The process of fermentation predigests the food and releases its nutrients, which makes them more accessible for our bodies to use. For example, sauerkraut has almost 20 times more bioavailable vitamin C in it than the same amount of fresh cabbage.[69] The famous British explorer James Cook, who discovered Australia and New Zealand, had barrels of sauerkraut on his ships to prevent scurvy in his crew.[68,69] Through the ages our physiology became used to having fermented food on a daily basis; it has become essential for us to stay healthy. Since we invented refrigeration, we humans have almost stopped consuming these foods. As a result, we are depriving ourselves of all the wonderful benefits that fermented foods would provide: probiotic bacteria to keep our gut flora healthy, easy-to-digest nutrients, active enzymes to keep us young and energetic and many other good things.

There are many easy fermentation recipes that you can use at home. You can find these recipes in many good books on nutrition and a few selected recipes in the recipe section of this book.

13. Drink freshly pressed fruit and vegetable juices

You will need to have a good juicer at home and buy fresh, organic fruit and vegetables to juice. It is important to use organic produce, because if you juice non-organic fruit and vegetables you will get concentrated amounts of pesticides and other agricultural chemicals in your glass of juice. Thousands of people all over the world have freed themselves from the most deadly diseases with juicing; dozens of books have been published on this subject, full of testimonies and hundreds of wonderful recipes.[86,87] Some very big names in natural medicine have strongly advocated juicing and used it actively in the treatment of their patients – people like Dr Max Gerson and Dr Norman Walker for example. Hundreds of scientific studies have been published on the health benefits of fresh raw fruit and vegetables. Juices provide all the goodness from these fruit and vegetables in a concentrated form and in large amounts. For example, to make a glass of carrot juice you need a pound of carrots. Nobody can eat a pound of carrots at once, but you can get all the nutrition from them by drinking the juice. The digestive system has virtually no work to do when digesting freshly pressed juices, they get absorbed in 20–25 minutes, providing the body with a concentrated amount of nutrients. With juicing you can consume large quantities of fresh vegetables and fruit every day in the most digestible and pleasant form.

Many children in our modern world will not eat fruit and vegetables, and I know quite a few adults like that as well. Juices, being so tasty, can provide an excellent solution to this problem. Drinking freshly extracted juice will provide you and your child with many essential vitamins, magnesium, selenium, zinc and other minerals, amino acids and lots more nutrients.[88,89] A combination of pineapple, carrot and a little bit of beetroot in the morning will prepare the digestive system for the coming meals, stimulate stomach acid production and pancreatic enzymes production. A mixture of carrot, apple, celery and beetroot has a wonderful liver-cleansing ability. Green juices from leafy vegetables (spinach, lettuce, coriander, parsley, dill, carrot and beet tops) with some tomato and lemon are a great source of magnesium and iron and can remove toxic metals from your body. Cabbage, apple and celery juice stimulates digestive enzyme production and is a great kidney cleanser. There is an endless number of healthy and tasty variations you can make from whatever organic fruit and vegetables you have available at home.[88,89,90] To make the juice taste nice, particularly for children, generally try to have 50% of less tasty but highly therapeutic ingredients – carrot, small amount of beetroot (no more than 5% of the juice mixture), celery, cabbage, lettuce, greens, such as spinach, parsley, dill, basil, fresh nettle leaves, beet tops, carrot tops – and 50% of some tasty ingredients: pineapple, apple, orange, grapefruit, grapes, mango, etc.

Any person with a degenerative disease, including atherosclerosis and heart disease, immune problems, neurological and psychiatric disorder, any person under a lot of stress, any person recovering from jet-lag or from an infection and any person who is run down or simply tired would benefit tremendously from drinking freshly pressed juices.[88,89]

What about fibre? Drinking juices doesn't mean that you stop eating fresh fruit and vegetables. You should carry on eating fruit and vegetables as usual. Treat the juices like a supplement of concentrated nutrients in a glass. They should be taken on an empty stomach 20–25 minutes before food and 2–2½ hours after a meal. Freshly pressed juices are highly perishable; they need to be consumed within a few minutes from extracting (30 minutes maximum). So, make just enough to be consumed immediately. Whatever has not been consumed can be frozen as ice lollies for children or ice cubes for making cold drinks later. Children, in particular, love freshly pressed juices. You can make smoothies for them by mixing the juice with mashed avocado or banana and adding it to yoghurt or home-made ice cream and sorbet.

But can't we just buy juices from shops? The answer is a big NO! Juices in the shops have been processed and pasteurised, which destroys all the enzymes and most vitamins and phytonutrients. They are a source of processed sugar, which will feed abnormal bacteria and fungi in the gut and upset your blood sugar level.[90] In freshly extracted juice the natural sugars are balanced with active enzymes, minerals, and other nutrients which turn them into nourishment and energy for the body. When you make your juice at home you know what you put into it, you know that it is fresh without any contamination or oxidation, and you can have great fun mixing different fruit and vegetables together to make different tasty combinations. There is a large number of books written on juicing with wonderful recipes for every health problem and every occasion.[86,87]

14. Beverages

We have already mentioned fermented beverages, such as good-quality wine and homemade kvass. We have also discussed freshly pressed juices. All these beverages are good for us in reasonable amounts.

Apart from those it is very important to drink plenty of water. What kind of water? As natural and as clean as possible and that, unfortunately, does not include tap water in many places of the world. Tap water contains many additives, which will absorb into your bloodstream and cause endothelial dysfunction: chlorine, fluoride, nitrates and agricultural chemicals to mention a few. That is why it is important to filter your tap water.

A lot of bottled water on the market is no better than your tap water. When buying bottled water, look for natural mineral water from an established and known producer, preferably in a glass bottle as plastic leaches a lot of chemicals into the water.[91,92,93,94,95] Lucky are those people who live near a clean well or a spring, where they can drink natural water without anything added to it. It is a good idea to add a slice of lemon or a teaspoon of organic apple cider vinegar to your glass of water, as they will add alkalising minerals and other good qualities.

Many of us like to have a hot beverage, such as tea or coffee. These drinks are stimulants and a lot of people get addicted to them without knowing it. The way to find out if you are addicted is to stop drinking coffee and tea for a few days. An addicted person will get serious headaches and cravings for these beverages. If you are not addicted to them, there is nothing wrong with having a cup of tea or a cup of coffee occasionally. But make sure that you have good-quality tea and coffee, freshly made out of quality organic ingredients, not instant and not processed.[96]

What you also have to understand is that coffee and tea are dehydrating for your body. This means that they make your body acid and very thirsty for water. Make sure that you rehydrate yourself with plenty of water and juicy fruit and vegetables at other times of the day. It will also help if you have your tea with a slice of lemon instead of milk and eat a good piece of juicy fruit with your cup of coffee. Replace sugar with honey and if you want a snack with your hot drink, a helping of natural nuts and dried fruit will remove many of the negative influences that coffee or tea may have on your body. Cheese and honey also make a good snack to have with your cup of tea or coffee. Make sure that the cheese is natural and made according to traditional practices. It goes without saying that you should avoid eating biscuits and cakes with your hot beverage, which unfortunately is exactly what people commonly serve.

There are many herbal teas on the market and their variety is growing. Most herbs are medicinal, which means that they will have a particular effect on your physiology. That is why many of them do not suit everybody. If you find a herbal tea that suits you, then make sure that it is organic, as non-organic herbal teas may contain heavy metals and other contaminants.[97,98]

It goes without saying that you must avoid all pop drinks and soft beverages, including cordials, if you want to avoid atherosclerosis and heart disease. They are made out of sugar and chemicals – a double toxic attack on your body.[99,100] The "sugar-free" soft drinks are even worse: they contain artificial sweeteners which can be even more toxic than sugar.[101,102]

Strong alcoholic beverages are something you may want to indulge in very occasionally and in very small amounts. They load your liver

with a lot of work, making it unable to handle the other toxins floating in your blood, which leaves them free to damage your endothelium. Excessive alcohol and its toxic by-products also directly cause
endothelial injury and dysfunction.[103]

A word of caution about beer: it is made from grains and in the
process of fermentation the starch from grain is broken down into various forms of carbohydrates. Beer is a concentrated source of processed
carbohydrates, which absorb quickly into your bloodstream and can
cause high blood sugar level and high insulin level. Both are dangerous, as they lay the ground for excessive weight gain, diabetes and
heart disease.[104] If you already have a predisposition to any of these
health problems it is a good idea to reduce your beer consumption or
to avoid it altogether.

In conclusion

We have discussed the first step that we need to take to avoid degenerative diseases, such as atherosclerosis and its complications, as well
as many others. It is probably the most important step, as 80–90% of
anything toxic that is floating in your blood comes from your digestive
system!

When feeding yourself or your family please remember these simple
rules:

Never economise on food!
Never compromise when it comes to food!
Because if you do not eat well, you will not be healthy, and if
you do not have your health, you will have no life!

Compromise and economise on clothes, cars, entertainment, toys, etc.,
etc., but never on food. Buy good quality and fresh food. Organic is
better than non-organic. Local produce is better than exotic food that
has had to travel half across the world. Fruit and vegetables grown in
a private garden are better than fruit and vegetables from any supermarket. Grass-fed animals are better than those raised on grains or
commercial animal foods. Traditionally grown and prepared food is
better than modern inventions. Pick your own berries, fruit and

vegetables whenever you have a chance. Prepare your food with love and care, do not burn or overcook it. Use traditional cooking methods, do not use microwave ovens. Those of you who make these simple changes will gain endless benefits.

Eating out a lot is a very unhealthy habit (that includes takeaway meals), because you have no idea what kind of ingredients and cooking methods were used to make your meal. So, make sure that most of what you eat is prepared at home.

Many people across the Western world have lost their sense of right or wrong where food is concerned. I will give you one example. I live in a small rural town in Britain. A lot of old houses here have mature apple trees in their gardens, which bring a prolific harvest of beautiful apples, full of minerals, vitamins, antioxidants, anti-cancer substances and other excellent nutrients. But people do not collect them because they think it is hard work. So, these wonderful gifts of Nature just fall to the ground and rot away while their owners buy their apples at the supermarket – apples that are nutritionally empty and full of agricultural chemicals. The children of these people grow up with the idea that it is all right to waste a wonderful food like that and eat a packet of crisps instead. This is just one example of how far away we are now from a natural way of living, which is the only way for us to stay healthy!

Step 2: Stop polluting your body!

Never go to a doctor whose office plants have died.

Erma Bombeck

We live in a polluted world. Every day we breathe in car fumes and industrial wastes. We eat foods containing pesticides, herbicides and other agricultural chemicals. We drink milk and eat meat from animals that are routinely given antibiotics, steroids and other drugs. We eat a countless number of various chemicals in processed foods. We use personal care products full of various chemicals shown to be carcinogenic and generally toxic for humans. Our modern energy-conserving homes and offices have become toxic places. Modern building materials, insulation, paints, domestic cleaning chemicals and fire retardants all outgas toxic substances, which we breathe day in and day out. For example, chemical analysis on the outgassing of common carpets and carpet adhesives in modern homes has found considerable amounts of toxic substances, such as formaldehyde, toluene, xylene, benzene, methacrylate, tetrachloroethylene, methyl naphthalene, phthalates and styrene.[1,2] All these chemicals are known toxins for humans and yet we breathe them in large quantities all the time we are at home. Hospitals and shopping centres have even higher amounts of toxic substances in the air, which is why many people feel so tired and drained after a shopping trip or a long visit to a hospital.[3] And as if all that is not enough, we routinely take prescription drugs, drink alcohol and smoke tobacco.

It is very easy to become disheartened when we start looking at the total toxic load our bodies have to carry in our modern world. However, there is a lot we can do to lighten that toxic load quite dramatically.

It is within our power to keep our houses as chemical free as possible by using minimal amounts of domestic cleaning chemicals, paints, carpet pesticides and other toxic substances. All widely available domestic chemicals are toxic.[4,5,16] Bathroom detergents, floor cleaners, polishes, etc. all stay in the air and on the surfaces, contributing to the general toxic load on your system. Toxic domestic chemicals can be replaced with safer biodegradable alternatives from various conscientious companies. However, try to use as few chemicals as possible. A lot of cleaning around the house can be done with water and a bit of vinegar or lemon juice, bicarbonate of soda and olive oil. You can clean your wood floors with strong tea. You can polish your furniture with a mixture of 1 cup of olive oil and ¼ cup of white vinegar. You can pour white wine on red wine spills on your carpet to remove the stain. There are many traditional natural ways of cleaning the house if you look for them.[6]

It is wise **not** to redecorate the house or install new carpets or furniture if you are ill or recovering from an illness. Paints, many building materials, new carpets and new furniture outgas a plethora of extremely toxic chemicals which we absorb through our lungs, skin and mucous membranes.[1,7,8,15,33,34] New carpet can outgas considerable amounts of highly carcinogenic formaldehyde for a few years. New furniture is full of fire retardants, which are great contributors of antimony (a toxic heavy metal) in our systems. Fresh household paints outgas dozens of extremely toxic chemicals into the air of the house for at least six months. Exposing yourself to these toxins will undermine your ability to recover from an illness and can make it worse.

Very important contributors to the general toxic overload in the body are *cosmetics, toiletries, perfumes and other personal care products.*[9,10] The personal care products industry uses more than a thousand of carcinogenic and toxic chemicals in the formulation of shampoos, soaps, toothpaste, cosmetics, perfumes, creams, deodorants, makeup, hair dyes, etc. The old belief that our skin is a barrier that does not let in toxins has proven to be completely wrong. Human skin absorbs most things from the environment very efficiently; in some cases even better than our digestive system.[9] The wide use of personal care products is a major contributor to our cancer epidemic.[10] Children, women and men are unknowingly exposing themselves to huge amounts of carcinogenic substances, which they apply to their skin. A good example is breast cancer. Cells removed from a cancerous breast, in many cases, are full of aluminium – a toxic metal.[11] Where does all this aluminium come from? Probably from deodorants, absorbed through the skin in the woman's armpits.

Many chemicals in personal care products and domestic cleaning formulas are synthetic oestrogens, which mimic the real oestrogens in our bodies, causing cancer of the breast, ovaries and other organs in women and infertility, impotence and other sexual abnormalities in men.[12,13,14] Recent research into toxic metals and other chemicals showed that when a pregnant animal is exposed to them they accumulate in large amounts in the foetus.[15,16] That is why it is particularly important for a pregnant or breast-feeding mother to be careful about what personal products and cosmetics she puts on her skin, face and hair; best to put none! Children and infants are particularly vulnerable to the toxic effects of these chemicals. And yet young mothers, who have just delivered their babies in maternity units in the United Kingdom, are given free bags full of colourful bottles of shampoos, bubble baths, baby lotions and other toiletries for the baby. All these products are full of toxins. A newborn baby and an infant should not have anything put on its skin apart from clean water!

The best substance to put on the nappy area is natural live yoghurt, sour cream or cold-pressed natural oil, such as olive oil, coconut oil, hemp oil, etc. It is no wonder that we have a growing epidemic of various cancers in our children. Apart from exposing children to cancer-causing toxins, soaps wash off protective oils from their skin, leading to eczema and other dry skin conditions.[17]

In this book we cannot go into the details of all the toxins present in our toiletries and cosmetics. But let us list some of the most common ones.

- Talc or talcum powder can cause ovarian cancer.[18] Do not use it, particularly on babies!
- Sodium Lauryl (Laureth) Sulfate (SLS) is a highly toxic detergent that is present in most shampoos, soaps and toothpaste. It is a cheap foaming agent and is used extensively by the personal care industry. It absorbs very effectively through mucous membranes and skin and causes endothelial injury, amongst many other damaging effects on the body.[19,20]
- Fluoride is a terrible poison for every system in the body. Widespread in toothpaste and other dental care products. It is added to some water supplies and given to babies as drops. If you are not familiar with its toxicity I would strongly advise you to learn more about it and avoid it like the plague. Fluoride accumulates in our bones and teeth undermining their structure. If you pay attention you will notice that a lot of people have white spots on their teeth (mottling of the teeth or fluorosis). This is accumulated fluoride which generally comes from toothpaste.[21]
- Titanium Dioxide is carcinogenic. It is present in many prescription drugs and personal care products.[22]
- Triethanolamine (TEA) and Diethanolamine (DEA) form carcinogenic nitrosamines in shampoos, makeup, soaps and some toothpaste. They are known to cause cancer of the liver and kidneys, as well as many other organs.[23]
- Lanolin, itself a non-toxic natural substance, is often contaminated with DDT and other carcinogenic pesticides.[24]
- Dioxanes are inhaled and absorbed through skin, they are highly carcinogenic and toxic for our immune system.[24]

- Saccharin – carcinogenic.[25]
- Formaldehyde in carpet adhesives, glue and household products is a toxic and carcinogenic substance. Apart from cancer it causes eye problems, skin rashes, allergies and respiratory problems.[24,33]
- Propylene glycol – extremely toxic and carcinogenic.[26]
- Lead, aluminium and other toxic metals are present in many personal care products, particularly in deodorants and makeup.[27]
- Hair dyes, particularly black and brown, contain DEA, TEA, ethoxy-lated alcohols, formaldehyde and other chemicals. Regular use of hair dyes would put you at risk of developing leukaemia, multiple myeloma, Hodgkin's disease and non-Hodgkin's lymphoma.[24]
- Fragrances in your perfumes, toiletries and cleaning products are very toxic and have been recognised as a considerable source of indoor air pollution. They absorb through our lungs and skin into the bloodstream and can cause atherosclerosis, cancer, neurological and psychiatric symptoms, allergies, sensitisation and many other health problems.[28]
- Sunscreens contain chemicals, which may cause skin cancer. Apart from that many of them contain synthetic oestrogens, such as benzophenone-3(Bp-3), homosalate (HMS), 4-MBC, OD-PABA and many others. They absorb through skin and can induce breast cancer, ovarian and uterine cancer, infertility in men and women, as well as abnormal and premature puberty in children.[29]

For a full list of harmful chemicals in toiletries and other personal care products, please read a very good book by Dr Samuel Epstein, MD, *Unreasonable Risk*.[24]

If we are to avoid falling prey to heart disease, atherosclerosis, cancer and many other maladies, our use of personal care products should be reduced to an absolute minimum. Your body does not need washing with soaps, shower gels or bubble baths. They not only contribute to the general toxic overload, but they also wash off important oils, which protect the skin from infections and drying out. Washing with water and a sponge is quite enough for us humans.

A child does not need any personal care products apart from natural toothpaste. There are a number of companies who produce safe personal care products without the harmful substances listed above.

Swimming pools are very toxic places.[29] People generally believe that going to a swimming pool is healthy exercise. This cannot be further from the truth. Apart from a few rare pools, sterilised with ozone, the rest use chlorine-based chemicals for sterilising the water. Chlorine is a poison, which affects every system in the body, particularly the immune system and the liver.[29,30] It absorbs quite well through the skin. Apart from that, a thick layer of chlorine gas floats above the swimming pool water, which children and adults inhale while swimming. Inhaled chlorine absorbs extremely well through the lungs into the bloodstream. Nature has designed us to swim in the natural waters of lakes, rivers and the sea instead of the toxic chemical soup of swimming pools. Natural waters are full of life, biological energy from plants and different creatures, minerals, enzymes and many other beneficial substances. Swimming in natural living waters has been prized as a therapy for many health problems for centuries.[31] Obviously, you have to make sure that the water you swim in is as far as possible from any source of industrial pollution.

Washing powders and liquids all stay in the fabric of our clothes, bedding and towels and also contribute to our toxic overload.[32] Try to look for safer ecologically friendly alternatives.

Houseplants are our great friends when it comes to keeping our houses toxin free. They consume the toxic gases and replace them with oxygen and other beneficial substances.

Try to reduce your exposure to electro-magnetic pollution and radiation. Do not walk around with your mobile phone constantly attached to your ear; use the phone only when you *really* need to. We have no solid data yet about what the radiation from mobile phones can do to us, but the preliminary data shows that it may put us at risk of developing a brain cancer.[32,37] Do not have TV sets, computers or any other electronic devices in your bedroom. When we sleep our bodies work hard to detoxify, to clean our blood and tissues, so give your body a chance to do that without adding more pollution. Try to limit your exposure to electronic screens and devices; spend more time in the fresh air instead. If your house is under a high voltage electricity line or close to a source of radiation or industrial pollution, then move to another area.

We have discussed just a few of the things you can do to reduce your exposure to man-made pollution. There is a mountain of information available on this subject. So, please research it and make changes in your life and your family's life to protect and improve your health.

One more thing to keep in mind!

One of the serious risk factors for heart disease and other complications of atherosclerosis is our attitude. People with tense and negative personalities get ill more often than people who have a more relaxed and happy attitude to life.[35] Why does that happen? Because every emotion creates a certain biochemistry in the body, and not just in your brain but everywhere else. Negative emotions create negative biochemistry, leading to disease. Positive emotions create positive biochemistry, leading to healing and recovery.

A few simple rules will help you to stay positive and hence create a positive biochemistry in your body.

1. Work to live, do not live to work! Workaholics are much more prone to heart attacks than people who keep their work in perspective. There are far more important things in life than earning money.
2. Remember what the little rabbit, called Thumper, said in the Disney film *Bambi*, "If you can't say something nice, say nothing at all!" Criticising other people and saying negative things about others will alter your own biochemistry and damage your own health.
3. Be positive! Concentrate on positive things in life, on your blessings, on your dreams, on the good qualities of people around you, on your own good qualities – and your life will become much happier as a result. That will create good biochemistry in your body. Concentrating on problems and bad things in life will poison your life and your biochemistry, bringing a disease with them.
4. Laughing can be extremely powerful in treating any disease. Actively create situations in life when you can laugh. Avoid situations that make you miserable. Seek the company of people who make you feel good and happy and avoid people who make you feel bad and low. Life is too short to spend it in bad company! If it is

your own company you enjoy the most, then create time for doing just that and make it happy.

5. Don't bottle up your feelings! Find a safe outlet for your anger, frustration and other destructive feelings. Don't hide grief; the more you share it with others the quicker it will leave you. Accumulated bad feelings destroy us from the inside.

6. Be honest with yourself and others. If your conscience is not clear, your biochemistry will be in a self-destructive mode and you will create a disease in your body out of nowhere.

7. Every single day organise yourself to do something that you really enjoy. Do it just for yourself. In doing that you will show yourself respect and love and that will create very positive, healing biochemistry in your body.

I would like to summarise with the words of the late Professor Christiaan Barnard, the world's most respected heart surgeon, who performed the world's first heart transplant operation: "I promise you: look after your soul and you will reduce your chances of a heart attack".[35]

What about exercise?

Everybody knows that exercise is good for you. Yet, the majority of us lead very physically inactive lives: sitting in offices all day, driving from door to door, sitting at home in front of the TV or the computer. Most of the time we are too busy to exercise or too tired. Then one day we suddenly remember about it and try to jog for miles or play an active sports game to the point of exertion. The usual results of this kind of exercise are aching joints, painful muscles and injuries. Having done that we go back to our inactive lifestyles. Sound familiar?

So, the question is, what kind of exercise is good for the heart? The answer is: any kind, as long as you enjoy it and do some of it consistently every day. *Moderate but consistent exercise is the best* for your heart and your overall health. If you have some goal to achieve, such as playing a sports game as well as you used to in your 20s, then start gradually and build up slowly. Throwing yourself in at the deep end is the worst thing you can do for your heart.

The most common reason for not exercising is lack of time. However, with a bit of planning everybody, even the busiest person, can incorporate some exercise into the daily routine. For example, you can walk or cycle to the office or shops instead of driving. Wherever you are going you can park further away from your destination and walk: even a few hundred metres walking will do you good. You can walk up the stairs instead of taking a lift. Getting a dog is one of the best things you can do for your heart: your dog will take you for a walk every day whether you like it or not. Walking in the fresh air is one of the best and most natural ways of exercising for us, humans.

Science has established that aerobic exercise is best for the heart.[36] Aerobic exercise makes you breathe much deeper and faster, it provides more oxygen for your body, it improves circulation and is generally very healthy. However, a very important point to keep in mind is that we must *breathe clean, fresh air when exercising.* Unfortunately, many gyms and other indoor sports areas do not provide clean, fresh air. Instead the air is full of cleaning chemicals, perfumes, disinfectants and other toxins. During exercise you breathe larger volumes of air than usual. If the air is full of toxins you draw large amounts of them into your body. It is best to exercise in the fresh air, rather than indoors, and to choose places away from man-made pollution. One clinical example demonstrates this point well: a 30-year-old marathon runner succumbed to lung cancer. She never smoked, she always exercised and tried to eat well. However, in the last few years she lived in London and every day she would run many miles along busy London roads in preparation for her marathons. The pollution that she pumped into her lungs while running probably caused her lung cancer.

Overweight and obese people need to be careful when it comes to exercise. Imagine attaching a large sack of potatoes to your body and trying to jog with it? Your heart and other organs and systems may not survive too long. This is what it is like for a seriously overweight person to exercise, and for an obese person vigorous exercise is positively dangerous. They should not do it! Change your diet first to lose weight, and when your body is ready it will give you a desire to start doing some exercise.

Find some form of exercise that suits you, fits into your busy day and that you really enjoy. *It is very important to enjoy your exercise!* The popular exercise mantra of "No pain – no gain!" will bring you only pain. If it is uncomfortable, painful and you are not particularly good at it, then don't do it! That kind of exercise will do you no good. We have all seen people jogging along the streets with pain and suffering on their faces. This kind of punishment exercise will create a lot of negative biochemistry in your body. Find something that is fun for you, that makes you feel good, makes you laugh, perhaps brings you new friends and makes your life fuller and happier.

Part Four: RELATED ISSUES, IMPORTANT TO KNOW

All diseases begin in the gut!
Hippocrates (460–370 BC)

The more we discover with all our modern science and the more we learn about human health, the more we realise just how right Hippocrates was! Our digestive system holds the roots of our health.[1,2] If we are to prevent or reverse atherosclerosis, heart disease and every other modern malady, we must take care of our digestive health! In order to do that we must take care of our gut flora.

What is gut flora?

Our planet is largely populated by microbes, they are everywhere including on the outside and the inside of our bodies. The vast majority of them are not only harmless for us humans, but beneficial.[1,2,3] In the process of evolution a symbiotic relationship has developed between microbes and the human body. Symbiotic means that we cannot live without each other! We need microbes to stay alive and healthy. They live on our skin, eyes and mucous membranes, as well as inside our bodies.[4,5] The largest colony of microbes lives inside our digestive system: an average adult carries 1,5–2,5 kg of bacteria in the gut.[4] These bacteria are not just a chaotic mass, but a highly organised microbial world. Certain species of bacteria predominate in the healthy digestive system and fulfil a number of functions, vital for the gut and the rest of the body.

We acquire our bodily flora, including our gut flora, at birth from our parents, mainly from the mother.[6] At the time of birth, as the baby goes through the birth canal, she swallows her first mouthfuls of bacteria. They settle in the baby's sterile digestive system and become her gut flora. At the same time microbes also populate the baby's skin and mucous membranes. The microbial flora in the birth canal comes from the mother's and father's bodily flora (mainly gut flora). So whatever lives in the parents' digestive systems will populate the baby's digestive system.[7] Babies who receive healthy gut flora from their parents are generally healthy babies. Unless antibiotics and other influences change their gut flora composition at some time, they will grow up to become adults with good strong constitutions.[7,8]

All microbes in the gut can be divided into three groups:

1. **Essential or beneficial flora.** These are the good bacteria, also called probiotic bacteria (probiotic means pro-life), beneficial yeasts and viruses and other beneficial creatures. They fulfil a myriad of vital functions in the body.[7,8] In a healthy person beneficial bacteria and beneficial yeasts predominate in the gut and control all other microbes. Unfortunately, they are very vulnerable when it comes to our modern drugs, particularly antibiotics.[9,10] Antibiotics damage beneficial bacteria, on average it takes these bacteria one to two months to recover. That gives other microbes a window of opportunity to grow and occupy parts of your digestive system. Once they are there it is very difficult to drive them out. Most other drugs, particularly when prescribed for long periods of time, damage your beneficial bacteria (painkillers, contraceptive pills, steroids, sleeping pills, neuroleptics, cholinolytics, cytotoxic drugs, etc.).[6,11,12,13] Drug-induced damage is usually the worst, but other modern influences can also damage your beneficial gut bacteria: processed foods, infectious diseases, prolonged stress, alcoholism, man-made chemicals, radiation, pollution, etc.[13]

2. **Opportunistic flora.** These are various bacteria, fungi, viruses and other microbes that are capable of causing serious health problems. Their numbers and characteristics vary in different individuals. In a healthy gut they live in small numbers and under tight control by the good bacteria, which will not allow them to do us any harm.[7,23,24] However, if the good bacteria are damaged or wiped out by antibiotics, steroids, other drugs and other influences, these opportunists get out of control and cause disease, not only in the gut but everywhere else in the body.[7,14,15] In fact, we carry many of our future health problems in our digestive systems right from the start of our lives, because we acquire much more from our parents than just genetics. Many diseases are passed through the genera-

tions via the bodily microbial flora, as the child acquires it from the parents. Autoimmune conditions, gout, predisposition to allergies, digestive problems, cancer and, of course, atherosclerosis and heart disease can be due to particular species of opportunistic microbes, which we received from mum and dad at birth.[16,17,18,19,20,21] However, as long as we take care of our beneficial bacteria, these opportunistic microbes may never show themselves.

3. **Transitional flora.** These are various microbes from the environment, which we swallow daily with our food and drink. If the gut is well protected by the beneficial flora these microbes usually do us no harm. However, if the beneficial microbes have been damaged then anything coming into your gut can harm you.

So, what does gut flora do for us and why do we need it?

The functions of beneficial gut microbes, currently known to science, are multiple and far reaching. Let us have a look at a few of them. So far scientists have largely studied only the beneficial bacteria and their functions in the body (hopefully the research on beneficial yeasts and viruses will follow).

1. *Probiotic bacteria are the housekeepers of our digestive system.* Without them your gut cannot be healthy. These bacteria coat the whole surface of the gut wall (from your mouth to the very end) providing a physical barrier to anything harmful. They produce antibiotics, antifungal and antiviral substances, which destroy any invader and control opportunists.[6,7,8] They chelate (in other words grab and keep hold of) mercury, lead, aluminium and other toxic metals, carcinogens and other toxic substances, preventing them from doing you any harm. The probiotic bacteria can destroy and neutralise many of these damaging things; those, that they cannot destroy, they hold tightly until they can be taken out of the system.[22] At the same time, these bacteria convert food into nourishing substances for the gut lining, feeding it and keeping it healthy.[25,26,27] If you have solid healthy gut flora, you will never develop digestive disorders including cancer in your digestive tract. When the beneficial bacteria get damaged, the gut wall deteriorates and becomes porous and leaky.[28] Substances, which normally

should not get through the gut wall, start getting through into the bloodstream and can cause hundreds of problems in the body. Undigested foods start autoimmunity and allergies, toxins cause headaches and block up your liver and kidneys, various microbes and parasites get from the gut into your blood.[29,30,31] Once in the blood, any of those harmful things can damage your endothelium, starting inflammation and the development of an atherosclerotic plaque.[19,20]

2. *Probiotic microbes are essential for feeding our bodies properly.* Without them normal digestion and absorption of food cannot happen. Not only do they ensure that your gut is healthy and in a good shape to digest food, but they also take an active part in the digestive process.[32,33] They produce a plethora of enzymes that break down proteins, carbohydrates, fibre and fats. They produce various substances that transport minerals, vitamins and other nutrients through the gut wall. And, as if that is not enough, they actively synthesise a number of nutrients that are essential for us: vitamin K2 (menaquinone), pantothenic acid, folate, thiamin (vitamin B1), riboflavin (vitamin B2), niacin (vitamin B3), pyridoxine (vitamin B6), cyanocobalamin (vitamin B12), various amino acids and other active substances.[32,33] In the process of evolution Nature made sure that when the food supply is sparse, we humans don't die from vitamin and amino acid deficiencies. Nature provided us with our own factory for making these substances – our healthy gut flora. And when this gut flora is damaged, despite adequate nutrition, we develop vitamin deficiencies. Why? Because many vitamins have a fairly short life in the body. So, unless one is taking these vitamins every hour (providing that they can be absorbed at all without healthy gut flora), there will be periods during the day when the body is deficient in these vitamins.[33] Remember that homocysteine, one of the most harmful chemicals for your endothelium, appears in the body when we are deficient in vitamins B6, B12 and folate.[34] Deficiency of vitamin K2 leads to deposition of calcium in the artery walls and atherosclerosis.[35] That is what happens to people with damaged gut flora, which is unable to provide a constant steady stream of these vitamins for the body to use. Restoring the beneficial bacteria in the gut is the best way to deal with those deficiencies.

After any injury your endothelium in the blood vessels has to heal itself. The healing process requires a plethora of nutrients: vitamins, minerals, amino acids, fats, etc. Without well-functioning gut flora you will develop deficiencies in those nutrients, and hence your body will not be able to heal any damage effectively. So, taking care of your gut flora means taking care of your endothelium and preventing atherosclerosis (as well as many other modern diseases).

3. *Gut flora is the right hand of our immune system.* Almost 85% of all our immunity is located in the gut wall, and the bacteria that live there play a crucial role in the proper functioning of our immune system.[36,37] There are many ways in which the gut flora influences our immunity. However, the first thing that happens to many people who lose beneficial bacteria in the gut is development of allergies. Why? Because our gut flora keeps two major arms of the immune system in the right balance (Th1 arm and Th2 arm). The Th1 arm is responsible for normal reactions to anything in the environment: dust, pollen, animals, foods, chemicals, etc. When the gut flora is damaged this arm becomes disabled. As a result the second arm Th2 tries to compensate for the disabled Th1 and becomes hyperactive. The Th2 arm is responsible for allergic (atopic) type reactions, so the person starts reacting to anything in the environment in an allergic way, developing hay fever, allergies to foods, animals, dust, etc.[38,39] Allergies cause a lot of damage in the body, including damage to your endothelium. As your immune system is in an unbalanced state, it will not deal with that damage appropriately leading to the development of an atherosclerotic plaque. Taking care of your gut flora is one of the most important things that you can do for your immune system!

How do we take care of our gut flora?

The interesting fact is that for millennia we humans used to take care of our gut flora daily without realising it: we used to ferment our foods. Until we invented refrigeration the best way to preserve food for long periods of time was fermentation. All year round every culture of the world consumed billions of probiotic microbes with fermented foods: yoghurts and cheese, sauerkraut, traditional (fermented) fruit and vegetable preserves, fermented fish and meats, fermented grains and beans, fermented beverages and condiments.[40,41,42] People in the Western world have largely lost the tradition of fermentation, which deprives us of probiotic microbes. There are excellent books with fermentation recipes that are easy to do at home. A few selected recipes are included in this book. They will help you to keep your gut flora healthy.

Apart from eating fermented foods you can take probiotic bacteria in the form of supplements. There is a plethora of probiotics on the market in different forms: powders, liquids, tablets and capsules. The food industry is producing more and more foods with added probiotic bacteria: drinks, snacks, etc., which are usually not as strong as the probiotic supplements. The majority of the supplements in the shops are prophylactic, which means they are designed for healthy people to maintain their gut flora. If you have any digestive problems or allergies then you need a therapeutic-strength probiotic with powerful species of beneficial bacteria.[43,44,45,46,47] In order to obtain one you may have to consult a qualified nutritionist.

Whatever you decide to do – take probiotic supplements or eat fermented foods – do it consistently. Taking care of your gut flora will save you from all sorts of modern diseases and maladies.

An obvious thing to do is to avoid inflicting damage to your gut flora. That means avoiding antibiotics and other drugs, particularly those prescribed for long periods of time. Obviously, there are situations when medication is absolutely necessary, but unfortunately a large percentage of prescriptions are not in that category. If you have to take antibiotics, then make sure that you eat fermented foods, such as *live* yoghurt and sauerkraut every day, and take a good-quality, therapeutic-strength probiotic. Continue for the duration of the antibiotic treatment and for a few weeks afterwards. Apart from medication, there are other influences that can damage your gut flora (which we have already discussed). Avoiding processed foods, man-made chemicals, radiation, pollution and other damaging influences will not only help you to keep your gut flora healthy, but prevent many modern diseases.

Your body functions as a whole. Everything in it is connected, interacting with each other and influencing each other. A well-functioning gut with healthy gut flora holds the roots of our health. And, just as a tree with sick roots will not thrive, the body cannot thrive without a well-functioning digestive system. The microbial population of the gut – the gut flora – is the soil around these roots, giving them their habitat, protection, support and nourishment. People with damaged gut flora become like plants with their roots pulled out of the soil: pale, limp and sick. So, take care of your roots! (To learn more about gut flora please read my book *Gut And Psychology Syndrome*).[48]

There is none so blind as the double blind!

We live in an age of 'evidence-based' medicine. What does it mean? It means that we medics cannot make one little step to the right, to the left, forwards or backwards until we have a stackful of double-blind, placebo-controlled studies to justify that step. The truth may be staring us in the face, our clinical knowledge and instincts may be telling us what to do, but we have to resist all that and say the famous phrase, "There is no evidence!" No evidence until Her Majesty Science provides us with that evidence. Let us have a look at her majesty and how much we can rely on her evidence.

It is amongst scientists that I meet the most cynical people, who do not believe anything. They have a good reason for that. They are the insiders, who know very well all the hundreds of different pitfalls in scientific studies. They also know all the hundreds of political knots our modern science is tied in. Science is an expensive business. Large numbers of studies are funded by companies or organisations that expect the scientists to come up with particular results to suit their agenda.[1,2] There are many ways of designing and conducting a scientific study that will ensure a particular result.[1,3,4] At the end of any study, when all the data is collected, it has to be statistically analysed. People who are familiar with statistics will tell you that there are many statistical methods for analysing the same data. Depending on which method you choose, you may arrive at very different results.[3,4] Large commercial companies, who conduct research to back their products, usually have an army of statisticians employed to do just that.[2,4] When the study is completed, the public at large is given a conclusion from that study, drawn by whatever party is interested in popularising that particular finding.[4,5] The public at large has no opportunity to look at the study in detail, to see the numbers and to interpret them for themselves. Of course, there are many properly conducted studies, but how do we know which one is which? The majority of people have no training, time or ability to analyse them. So, people are fed the "scientific evidence", based on studies that are often politically manipulated, statistically twisted or simply incorrectly conducted.

There is no other science so thoroughly confused and confusing than nutritional science. Incidentally, it is amongst nutritional scientists that I meet a lot of very unhealthy people. They are the people who tell us what we should and should not eat, so they should be healthy themselves, shouldn't they?

The majority of nutritional scientific studies are funded by the food industry.[1,4,5] Is it a surprise then that all the brightly packaged foods offered to us by the food industry are fully backed by nutritional science? Foods with virtually no nutritional value, full of E-numbers, flavour enhancers, colorants, preservatives, chemically altered proteins, chemically altered fats and carbohydrates, pumped with sugar and salt. Never in the course of human civilisation have there been such drastic changes in the way we eat as in the last 60–70 years. Apart from the food industry, who else do we have to thank for this change? The humble nutritional science, of course, which has provided us with huge amount of confusion and misinformation about foods. Their "scientific evidence" made us abandon the natural foods that we have eaten for thousands of years, and replace them with nicely packaged chemical concoctions, which we call "food" nowadays. There is no doubt that these dramatic changes in the way we eat are largely responsible for the epidemics in obesity, diabetes, heart disease, cancer and many other health problems, which plague the human race today.

For every bunch of nutritional studies telling you that a particular food or nutrient is harmful for you, one can find an equal number of studies telling you how good it is for you. I would certainly never rush to make any conclusions based on one study. But unfortunately that is exactly what happens.[3,4]

I will never forget a presentation made by the head clinical nutritionist of one of the top kidney hospitals in the United Kingdom. After an hour of listening to all the scientific evidence available on the subject, the audience was completely confused about what the right nutritional management of patients with kidney failure should be. It was obvious that the nutritionist, charged with helping these patients, was thoroughly confused as well. The audience went home feeling very sorry for the patients of that kidney hospital.

It is particularly amusing to see scientists proclaiming what we should or should not eat based on studying one particular small aspect of human biology. A lot of worried parents of autistic children once contacted me to say that a scientist in a seminar had told them that olive oil is bad for their children. This earth-shattering advice was based on a study of one particular chemical reaction in the body, where one of the ingredients of olive oil apparently may be interfering with that particular chemical reaction. Well, a human body is not equal to that one chemical reaction; it has trillions of chemical reactions going on at the same time, interacting with each other, changing in response to what the body is doing at the time and many other factors. Olive oil is not made from one ingredient either. It has dozens of different ingredients and, as a whole, is a time-proven health-giving food, used by people for thousands of years. But, of course, that scientist had spent years studying that one chemical reaction, so naturally that was the most important single issue in the whole of the human body, as far as this scientist was concerned. If you spend long enough digging a hole in the ground, then your whole world becomes that hole.

In our modern world it is very easy to become a victim of "scientific evidence". Of course, those scientists have laboratories and expensive and sophisticated equipment, so they should know! I meet patient after patient confused and bewildered by all the conflicting bits of information they get from different scientific sources. As a result, they finish up at a complete loss about what exactly they should eat and what they should not.

People are absolutely right to try and learn as much as possible. The more you know, the more you are able to help yourself. However, there are a number of things which are important for you to realise before looking at the scientific evidence.

- Scientific evidence is often full of conflicting information that negates itself. So, unless you have thoroughly ploughed through every study on the subject, do not attempt to make any conclusions.
- Science is tightly bound by political and commercial constraints, so never take any single study at its face value.
- An amazingly large percentage of studies are conducted or interpreted incorrectly.
- Science can only present you with what it has studied. It cannot tell you anything about things that it hasn't got round to studying yet.

As a result, that little bit of knowledge may give us a completely wrong view of the whole problem. A little knowledge is more dangerous than no knowledge at all.

- Scientific evidence can only be used in the context of proper clinical assessment of the patient, and must never be taken as gospel on its face value.

Scientific evidence is like a large jigsaw puzzle, where each study is a small piece. Because not all aspects of the problem have been studied yet, an unknown number of pieces of this puzzle are missing. On top of that, many available pieces may be false and misleading. God save anybody who tries to manage their health based on this puzzle!

So, what are we to do?

I am not on a crusade against science! It is thanks to science we, humans, have reached such a high level of sophistication. Because we have made science work for us! It is our human ideas, ethics, instincts, empirical knowledge and experience that employed the science and used it to our advantage. Not the other way round! At the moment, we have a situation where we are afraid to think or to listen to our instincts or experience unless science allows us to. From being our employee, science has become our boss. Remember, that it is our human mind that has to put all the pieces of the scientific jigsaw puzzle in the right places. Without that they mean nothing.

It is the human mind that employs experience, empirical knowledge, thinking and available scientific data and thus creates progress. Throughout the years there have always been doctors and other medical practitioners whose clinical experience and knowledge has led them against the scientific evidence available at the time. Health practitioners, who work with real people every day, dealing with their real health problems, accumulate an empirical clinical knowledge of what works and what doesn't. These people are not working with laboratory equipment, detached from patients. Very often their clinical experience goes against perceived science. But more often than not, science eventually confirms what these people knew through their clinical experience all along. Unfortunately, this kind of medicine does not fit into the straightjacket of 'evidence-based', official medicine.[4] As a result, more often than not, the official medicine brands it quackery and alternative. It is no secret that official Western medicine is run by the pharmaceutical industry, where money and profit rule the roost.[4,6] Alternative medicine uses diet and natural ways of healing the patient. There is no profit in that for the pharmaceutical industry, so this rather powerful industry does not like alternative medicine.

Where does all this leave the patient? Well, millions of patients around the world have discovered that, having been through every expensive test and treatment of the evidence-based, very scientific official medicine, they obtain real help from using diet and natural approaches. There is centuries-old wisdom that has been accumulated in treating disease with natural means. A lot of modern scientific knowledge has complemented and confirmed this wisdom. It is an area where science knows its place.

To conclude, we should not become intimidated by scientific evidence and should never try to make any changes in our lives based just on it. Science is only one of the tools in our human toolbox. Let's keep it in its right place!

Conclusion

Mother Nature gave us perfect bodies – miraculous creations, which we probably will never fully understand. Our bodies have complete power to keep themselves healthy, to repair any damage and heal themselves. It is your own body that heals you, not your doctor! It does it quietly without your knowledge as long as you allow it to do so.

Every time you put processed food in your mouth and expose yourself to pollution you give your body a message:

I do not respect you!
I do not love you, and
I do not care for you!

This kind of message will have far-reaching consequences for your health – both physical and mental!

Unfortunately, a large percentage of the Western population gives exactly that message to their bodies every day. We pollute our bodies with processed foods and myriads of chemicals and we use and abuse our bodies with our modern self-indulgent life styles. When the body becomes ill from this abuse, it starts calling for help: so you get pain, stiffness, inflammation and other symptoms. This is the only way that the body can let you know that it is in danger, that you are doing something wrong to it. But, instead of listening, we go to the doctor and get drugs to stop the pain, to stop the inflammation and to stop other symptoms. All these drugs do is to tell the body: "Stop calling for help and suffer in silence!", so we can go on destroying our health without being aware of it.

Someone clever once asked: "If you destroy your body, where are you going to live?"

Nature will always win. As we, humans, conquered epidemics of infectious disease, we replaced them with epidemics of man-made degenerative diseases. Heart disease, atherosclerosis, cancer and other maladies kill more people per year than any infection ever did. We created these epidemics ourselves by adulterating our food and polluting our bodies with man-made poisons.

But let us be positive. We live in a wonderful world of freely available information and an abundance of choices we can make. Good health is our birthright! Let us keep that right firmly in our own hands by keeping well-informed and making correct choices!

Selected Recipes

The recipes in this section are not designed to be glamorous. They are designed to introduce you to a wholesome, healthy way of cooking on a daily basis. You can always adapt your favourite recipes to the principles discussed in this book by replacing processed ingredients with natural healthy ones. Most recipes in this book will serve approximately four people.

Fermented foods

Fermented dairy
Yoghurt, kefir and sour cream (crème fraiche)
Fermented flour products
Russian pancakes
Sourdough bread
Fermented probiotic beverages
Kefir whey
Beetroot kvass
Kvass from other fruit and vegetables
Probiotic tomato juice
Fermented vegetables
Sauerkraut
Vegetables fermented with kefir or yoghurt culture
Vegetable medley
Fermented fish
Fermented herring or mackerel
Fermented sardines

Fats for cooking

Ghee
Goose or duck fat
Pork, lamb or beef fat
Coconut oil

Soups

How to make meat stock: Lamb, pork, beef or game stock
Chicken stock
Fish stock
Basic soup recipe
Spring nettle soup
Russian Borsch
Fish soup
Meatball soup
Beautiful winter squash soup
Meat jelly (brawn)

Salads

Beetroot salad
Tuna salad
Salad with cabbage and apple
Salad with tomatoes and cucumber
Russian salad
Carrot salad

Main dishes

Italian meat casserole
Stuffed peppers
Meatballs
Meat cutlets
Fish cutlets
Marinated wild salmon
Swedish gravlax
Baked beans or French cassoulet
Liver pudding
Liver in a clay pot
Quick liver recipe
Baked vegetables

Baking at home

Basic bread/cake/muffin recipe

Desserts

Baked apples
Crème caramel
Apple crumble
Apple pie
Winter squash cake
Cake Pinocchio
Peanut butter pie
Russian custard
Apple sauce
Birthday cake

FERMENTED FOODS

Fermented dairy: yoghurt, kefir and crème fraiche

You can buy live yoghurt, live kefir and crème fraiche from many shops. If you would like to make your own at home, here are the recipes.

I strongly recommend using only organic milk: cow's, goat's or sheep's, whichever you prefer. A lot of milk on the supermarket shelves, apart from being pasteurised, has been subjected to a process, called homogenisation in order to stop milk from separating in the bottle. This process breaks down the fat globules and changes the structure of milk even further, making it harmful for the body. Try to buy organic milk, which has not been processed at all. If it is not possible to buy unpasteurised milk, try to buy milk that has not been subjected to any other processing other than pasteurisation.

Goat's yoghurt is much more liquid than cow's yoghurt. You can use it as a drink or, if you want to thicken it, you can drip it through cheesecloth.

To make yoghurt you need to introduce bacteria into the milk. You can buy commercially available yoghurt starters from many health food shops or small holding suppliers. Alternatively, you can use commercially available *live* yoghurt as a starter. After making their first batch of yoghurt, many people successfully perpetuate their own yoghurt by using it as a starter for the next batch. You can also keep the liquid left from dripping your yoghurt, called the whey, in a clean, dry jar in your refrigerator to use as a starter for making the next batch of yoghurt. If, at any point, your own yoghurt or the whey does not work, you need to start again with a commercial starter or commercial live yoghurt.

For many patients I recommend using a variety of yoghurt called kefir. Apart from good bacteria a healthy body is populated by beneficial yeasts, which normally protect the person from pathogenic (bad) yeasts, such as the candida family. Kefir contains these beneficial yeasts (as well as the beneficial bacteria), which makes it very effective in people with an overgrowth of yeast in their bodies.

Instructions for making kefir and yoghurt

1. If you are using pasteurised milk in a stainless steel pan, bring 1 litre of milk (goat's or cow's) close to boiling, stirring occasionally. You need to bring the milk close to boiling point in order to destroy any bacteria, which may linger in the milk and interfere with the fermentation. However, do not boil the milk, as it will change its taste. Take the pan off the heat. Cover the pan with the lid. Cool by placing the pan into cold water until the temperature of the milk is around 38–45°C (100–118°F). If you do not have a suitable thermometer use your hand to determine the right temperature. Take a teaspoon of milk from the pan (using a clean, dry spoon) and put the milk on the inside of your wrist. If it feels just slightly warm, then the temperature is right. If you are using raw organic milk, which has not been pasteurised or processed in any other way, you don't need to heat it, so just skip this step.

2. If you are using a commercial kefir or yoghurt starter in powder form you need to dissolve the powder in a little milk first before adding it to the pan. If you are using your own kefir, yoghurt or commercial live kefir or yoghurt, add 1/3 cup to the milk. Stir well, cover with the lid and put in a warm place, preferably at 38–45°C (100–118°F). You can use a clean, dry thermos for this purpose, or a

yoghurt maker, an electric plate, the top of your boiler or your airing cabinet (if it is warm enough). Ferment the kefir or yoghurt for 12–24 hours, or until it reaches the right consistency.

3. After the fermentation is complete, move your kefir or yoghurt into a clean, dry glass jar, cover and refrigerate.
4. To drip the kefir or yoghurt line a large colander with a double layer of cheesecloth. Place the colander in a large bowl and pour your yoghurt into the lined colander. Cover with a tea towel and let it drip for a few hours. **Whey** is a clear, yellow liquid, which drips out through the cloth. Diluted with water or any freshly pressed juice, it makes an excellent probiotic beverage. You can use it as a starter for fermenting other foods (if you are allergic to dairy use juice from sauerkraut or the vegetable medley as a starter). Put whey into a clean, dry glass jar and keep it refrigerated. It will keep for a very long time without reducing its potency (up to a year). Depending on how long you leave your yoghurt dripping, you can make a soft cottage cheese or thicker yoghurt. Both soft cottage cheese and the yoghurt or kefir can be used for baking, adding to salads and soups and as desserts with honey and fruit.

Instructions for making sour cream (crème fraiche)
By using cream instead of milk you can make crème fraiche, or soured cream. For 1 litre of cream use one sachet of commercial starter, or 1 cup of live kefir or yoghurt.

1. Constantly stirring, bring the cream to the boil but do not let it boil. Skip this step if you are using organic raw cream (not pasteurised or processed in any other way).
2. Cool by placing the pan in cold water. Keep the pan covered at all times.
3. Test the temperature; it should be 38–45°C (100–118°F).
4. Add the starter and ferment for 24 hours minimum.

This soured cream, or crème fraiche, is very nice to use in salads, soups and stews, in baking or as a dessert with some honey and berries. You can blend it with a little honey and frozen fruit or berries to make an instant ice cream.

Fermented flour products

Before our food industry transformed itself about 70–80 years ago and changed the way we eat, for thousands of years people ate flour products only in a fermented form, because they knew that flour made out of grains is difficult to digest. Grains contain phytates, lectins and other damaging substances, while the nutrients in them are locked up in such a way that our human digestive system cannot access them. The fermentation process predigests the flour, releases vitamins, minerals and other nutrients from it and adds enzymes and probiotic bacteria to the finished product. Food made out of fermented flour is easy to digest for infants and the elderly and even for people who are allergic to wheat. Making bread by using fermentation with lactic acid bacteria, as well as yeast, makes it much tastier and allows it to keep for a long time. In fact the longer you keep it, the more the bread matures. The modern practice of using baker's yeast for bread making produces bread that spoils quickly and does not have the same nutritional qualities. Women in Europe, Russia and America used to have a pot of sourdough starter in their kitchens, so they could make bread, cookies and muffins any time they wanted. Sourdough is made with a natural mixture of lactic acid bacteria (probiotic bacteria) and beneficial yeasts. In fact, all natural fermentation is initiated by yeasts, which have an ability to break down hard-to-digest substances in grains. Once the yeasts have done their job, the lactic acid bacteria take over and complete the fermentation process.

Traditional Russian pancakes (blini)

500g (1.1lb) organic strong stone-ground white flour (wheat)
2 cups (250ml) whey
6 eggs
1 teaspoon sea salt
3–4 tablespoons ghee (or coconut oil, butter, goose fat, duck fat, pork fat, etc.)
a block of good-quality unsalted butter (for putting on made pancakes)

In a large glass bowl mix the flour and whey thoroughly. If it is too thick add water to reach the consistency of a thick soup. If there are lumps put the mixture through a sieve to break them down. Cover the bowl with a cotton towel and put into a warm place to ferment for 24–36 hours.

Separate the yolks and whites of the eggs into separate bowls. Whip the yolks until thick and pale. Whip the whites until stiff.

Gently mix the yolks and salt into the dough. Now gently fold the whites into the mixture. Finally add melted ghee and mix well.

Cook in a frying pan (stainless steel with a thick bottom) or a cast iron skillet. At the beginning you will need to grease the pan with ghee (or any other listed fat). After the first pancake the ghee in the mixture will keep the pancakes from sticking. Make the pancakes as thin as possible.

Melt the block of butter in a separate pan over a gentle heat. When each pancake is ready, transfer it to a plate and smear it with plenty of melted butter. The butter will soak into the pancake (while it is hot), making it soft and juicy, so it will be delicious to eat hot or cold.

You can eat these pancakes with jam or honey. Traditionally, Russians spread each pancake with honey, then roll it up and dip it into melted butter before taking a bite. Serve with tea.

You can also eat these pancakes with savoury fillings, such as cooked minced meat, smoked salmon, tuna mix (tinned tuna with onion and mayonnaise), chopped hard boiled eggs, chutney, pieces of cooked meat or cooked fish, etc. In Russia people traditionally fill them with caviar.

Sourdough bread

(Recipe from *Nourishing Traditions* by Sally Fallon)
Before making the bread you have to make the sourdough starter.

Sourdough starter

Makes about 3½ litres (3 quarts)
2 cups freshly ground rye flour
2 cups (500ml) cold filtered water
cheesecloth
6 cups freshly ground rye flour
cold filtered water

The best results for sourdough starter are obtained from rye rather than wheat flour, perhaps because rye contains lower phytates content than wheat. You will need two 4½ litre- (1 gallon-) sized bowls. The total time to make the starter is 1 week.

Grind 2 cups flour and let it sit for a bit to cool. In one large bowl, mix flour with 2 cups of cold water. The mixture should be quite soupy. Cover with a double layer of cheesecloth secured with a rubber band – this will allow yeasts and bacteria to get in but will keep insects out. In warm weather, you may set the bowl outside in the shade if you live in an unpolluted area and no pesticides have been used in your garden. Otherwise, keep it in a warm open area indoors or on a patio.

The next day and every day for a total of 7 days, transfer the starter to the other clean bowl and add 1 cup freshly ground rye flour plus enough cold water to make a soupy mixture. Cover and let stand. After a few days the starter will begin to bubble and develop a wine-like aroma. It should go through a bubbly, frothy stage and then subside. After 7 days, the starter is ready for breadmaking. Use 3 litres (2 quarts) for a batch of sourdough bread but save 1½ litre (1 quart for your next batch of starter. If not using the remaining starter immediately, you may store it in airtight jars in the refrigerator or freezer.

Do not be tempted to add honey to your starter, as some recipes require. Honey encourages the proliferation of yeasts at the expense of lactic-acid producing bacteria and may give you an alcoholic fermentation.

To start a new batch of starter, place the 1½ litre (1 quart) of leftover starter in a clean bowl. Add 1 cup freshly ground rye flour plus water each day, changing bowls, until 3½ litres (3 quarts) are obtained.

Sourdough bread

Makes 3 large loaves or 5–6 smaller loaves
3 litres (2 quarts) sourdough starter
13 cups freshly ground spelt, kamut or hard winter wheat
2 ½ tablespoons coarse sea salt
about 1½ cups cold filtered water

Traditional sourdough bread, prepared with a starter rather than with yeast, has a delicious flavour but tends to be heavy for modern tastes. Spelt gives the most satisfactory loaf.

Your starter should be at room temperature and have gone through the bubbling, frothy stage.

Place starter, salt and 1 cup water in a large bowl and mix with a wooden spoon until the salt crystals have dissolved. Slowly mix in the flour. Towards the end you will find it easier to mix with your hands. You may add the other ½ cup of water if the dough becomes too thick. It should be rather soft and easy to work. Knead by pulling and folding over, right in the bowl, for 10 to 15 minutes; or knead in batches in your food processor.

Without pressing down the dough, cut or shape loaves into the desired shapes or place into 3 large well-buttered loaf pans or 5–6 smaller loaf pans. Cut a few slits in the top of the dough, cover and let rise from 4 to 12 hours, depending on the temperature. Bake at 180° (350°F) for about an hour. Allow to cool before slicing.

The bread will keep for up to a week without refrigeration.

Variation: Sourdough Herb and Nut Bread
To each loaf, add 1 tablespoon rosemary or 1 tablespoon dill during kneading and ¼ cup chopped crispy pecans or walnuts at the end of the kneading process.

Variation: Sourdough Cheaters Bread
Use 3 cups unbleached white flour and 10 cups whole wheat flour for a lighter loaf.
(Recipe courtesy of Sally Fallon)

Fermented probiotic beverages

Using whey as a starter you can make delicious fermented beverages for the whole family. They will provide you with beneficial bacteria, enzymes and many nutrients, which the fermentation process will release from the fruit and vegetables. **If you are allergic to dairy, use a commercial yoghurt or kefir starter or some juice from the sauer-kraut or the vegetable medley** (see the recipe).

Yoghurt or kefir whey

The clear, yellow liquid left after dripping your yoghurt or kefir is called whey. It is a very nourishing beverage and an excellent source of probiotic bacteria. You can add it to freshly pressed juices, soups and stews. You can add salt and spices to it and drink the whey as it is, or diluted with some water. You can use it as a starter for fermenting vegetables, fruit, fish and grains.

Beetroot kvass

Using a knife finely slice medium-size beetroot. Don't grate the beet-root in a food processor as that destroys the beetroot and will make it ferment too quickly, producing alcohol. Put the beetroot into a 2-litre jar, add 1–2 tablespoons good-quality sea salt, 1 cup whey, 5 cloves garlic, 1 teaspoon freshly grated ginger (optional) and fill up with water. Let it ferment for 2–5 days in a warm place. Then keep in the refrigerator. Drink, diluted with water. Keep topping the water up in the jar to keep your kvass going for a long time. When it starts getting pale, the beetroot is spent. Take the beetroot out and replace with a fresh one.

Kvass from other fruit and vegetables

You can make kvass from any combination of fruit, berries and vegeta-bles. Try to experiment. Another good recipe is apple, ginger and rasp-berry kvass. Slice a whole apple, including the core, grate ginger root (about a teaspoonful) and get a handful of fresh raspberries. Put them all into a 1-litre jar, add ½ cup whey and top up with water. Let it brew for a few days at room temperature, then keep in the refrigerator. Drink diluted with water. Keep topping up your brew with water until the fruit is spent, then start again.

Probiotic tomato juice

Blend well 1 cup whey, 1–2 tablespoons tomato puree, 1 cup water and some salt to taste.

Fermented vegetables

Sauerkraut

Sauerkraut is a fermented white and/or red cabbage, commonly consumed in Germany, Russia and Eastern Europe. It is a wonderful healing remedy for the digestive tract, full of digestive enzymes, probiotic bacteria, vitamins and minerals. Eating it with meats will make them more digestible, as the sauerkraut has a strong ability to stimulate stomach acid production. For people with low stomach acidity I recommend having a few tablespoons of sauerkraut (or juice from it) 10–15 minutes before meals. For children, initially add 1–3 tablespoons of the juice from the sauerkraut to their meals.

Thinly slice medium-size white cabbage and add 2 shredded carrots. You can use red cabbage or a mixture of white and red. Add salt to taste: about 1–2 heaped tablespoons per medium-size cabbage. Knead the mixture well with your hands until a lot of juice comes out. Pack the mixture into a suitable glass bowl. Press it very firmly to get rid of any trapped air until the cabbage is drowned in its own juice. Place a plate, which is about 1cm smaller in diameter than the bowl, on top of the cabbage. The gap will allow the fermentation gases to escape. On top of the plate place something that is heavy enough to keep the cabbage constantly submerged in its juice. Cover the bowl with a kitchen towel to keep the mixture in the dark. It should take about 7–14 days inside a warm house for the sauerkraut to be ready. It will take two weeks in a cool place, like a garage. When the sauerkraut is ready skim off any cabbage on the top that may have gone dry, and throw it away. The rest of the cabbage will have a tangy, healthy smell and taste. Once ready, pack the sauerkraut into glass jars, making sure that the cabbage is submerged in its own juice and cover tightly. Store the jars in a cold place. It will keep refrigerated, or in any other cold place, for at least a year. Sauerkraut is delicious with any meal and it can be added to your home-made soups and stews.

Using this method you can ferment any vegetable or a mixture of vegetables. Just make sure that you add salt at the beginning and knead well with your hands so a lot of juice comes out. The reason for this is that during the fermentation process the vegetables must be completely covered by their own juice. If they are dry, they will rot. So, if any vegetable you are using is not very juicy, you may add a little bit of water until it is completely covered with liquid. It is essential to add salt at the beginning because the salt will stop any bad bacteria growing until the good ones start producing lactic acid, which will take over from the salt and stop any rotting. Experiment with your own mixtures and combinations, add natural spices, aromatic seeds (such as coriander, cumin, dill, fennel seeds, etc.), cranberries and fresh herbs.

Vegetables fermented with kefir or yoghurt culture

Using kefir or yoghurt whey, or the commercial starter, you can ferment vegetables. Take some cabbage (white, red or any other variety), beetroot, garlic, cauliflower and carrot and slice them into bite-size pieces, or shred them roughly. Add some salt to taste and pack loosely into a 1-litre glass jar. Dissolve the contents of the starter sachet in ½ litre of cold water. Alternatively, add ½ cup of your kefir or yoghurt whey to the water. Add this water to the jar until it completely covers the vegetables. It is important that the vegetables are completely covered by the water because if they are left dry at the top they will get mouldy. Cover tightly with the lid and leave to ferment at room temperature for a week. These vegetables, and the liquid that they ferment in, are an excellent probiotic food and will assist digestion. Eat them as pickles with your meals.

Vegetable medley

This probiotic food will provide you with delicious fermented vegetables and a wonderful beverage to drink, full of great nutrition and beneficial bacteria. In a 5-litre stainless steel pan put a whole cabbage, roughly cut, a medium-size beetroot, sliced, a handful of peeled garlic cloves and fresh dill or coriander. The pan should be half filled with the vegetables. Add 2 tablespoons of good-quality sea salt, 1 cup of kefir or yoghurt whey and top up with water until the pan is full. Float a small plate on top of the brine to keep the vegetables completely submerged, because if the vegetables are dry at the top they will get mouldy. Leave to ferment for 1–2 weeks at room temperature. When ready the vegetables will be soft and tangy. To stop fermentation move the pan into the refrigerator. You can add these vegetables to your soups and stews, drink the brine diluted with water with your meals or between meals and eat the vegetables with the meats. When the brine and the vegetables start getting low, add fresh cabbage, beetroot, garlic and some salt, top up with water and ferment at room temperature again. To this vegetable medley you can add a few florets of cauliflower, sliced carrot, Brussels sprouts and broccoli. You can keep this vegetable medley going forever, as long as you keep feeding it with more fresh vegetables. The brine from this medley is an excellent remedy for any tummy upset, food poisoning, sore gums and sore throat.

Fermented fish

Fermented herring or mackerel

3–4 very fresh large herrings or mackerel
1 small white onion
1 tablespoon peppercorns (black, red or a mixture)
5–7 bay leaves
1 teaspoon coriander seeds
fresh dill or some dill seeds
2 tablespoons salt per litre of brine
1 cup kefir or yoghurt whey
a suitable size glass jar

Skin the fish, remove the bones and cut into bite-size pieces. Peel and slice the onion. Place the pieces of fish in the glass jar and mix with peppercorns, slices of white onion (optional), coriander seeds, bay leaves and dill seeds or dill herb. In a separate jug dissolve the salt in some water and add ½ cup of kefir whey. Pour this brine into the jar until the fish is completely covered. If the fish is not covered, just add more water. Close the jar tightly and leave to ferment for 3–5 days at room temperature, then store in the fridge. Serve with vegetables, fresh dill, spring onion and some mayonnaise. Consume within 1–2 weeks.

Fermented sardines

5–7 very fresh sardines
1–2 tablespoons salt
1 tablespoon peppercorns
5–7 bay leaves
1 teaspoon coriander seeds
fresh dill or some dill seeds
1 cup kefir or yoghurt whey
a suitable size glass jar

Descale the fish, cut off the heads and clean out the belly. Put into a suitable size glass jar or a stainless steel pan. Add all the other ingredients. Top up with water so the fish is completely covered. You may want to float a small plate on top of the fish to keep it submerged in the brine. Cover the pan, or put the lid on the jar, and let it ferment for 3–5 days at room temperature. When the fish is ready take the meat off the bones, cut into bite-size pieces and serve with new potatoes, fresh dill and some chopped red onion.

FATS FOR COOKING

Cooking (roasting, frying, etc.) should be done with animal fats and fully saturated fats, because these fats generally do not alter their chemical structure when heated. The best fats for cooking are: pork dripping, goose fat, duck fat, lard, lamb fat, beef fat, coconut oil, butter and ghee. You can purchase many of these fats in shops and from traditional butchers. It is also easy to make many of these fats at home, which has an advantage: you know exactly what is in them.

Ghee

Ghee is a clarified butter. It is traditionally used in many cultures around the world for cooking and baking. Butter can be used for cooking very effectively. However, small amounts of whey in the butter often burn. Ghee on the other hand does not contain any whey, just milk fat, and does not burn.

Preheat your oven to around 100–120°C (250°F). Put a large block of organic, unsalted butter into a metal dish or pan. Leave it in the oven for 45–60 minutes. Take the pan out and carefully pour the golden fat from the top (ghee), making sure that the white liquid at the bottom stays in the pan. Discard the white liquid. Keep the ghee in glass jars and refrigerate.

Goose or duck fat

Roast a goose or a duck in the oven in the usual way. Take the bird out and pour the fat through cheesecloth or a fine metal sieve. Keep in glass jars and refrigerate. Use for cooking meats and vegetables. These fats give a nice flavour to roasted vegetables in particular and are known in traditional cultures to have health-protective qualities. People in those areas of France where foix gras comes from have a very low incidence of heart disease; traditionally they eat a lot of duck fat.

Pork, lamb or beef fat (lard)

You can collect these fats in much the same way as the duck and goose fats. You need any bits of fat from the animal. It is particularly good to use the internal fat layer from the animal, which butchers often sell very cheaply. You will be amazed by how much cooking fat you will collect from a fairly small piece. It is wise to use organic animals for this purpose, as fat is a natural body storage for various toxins. Investing in a small piece of organic fat once or twice a year will not cost you much and will last for many months.

Roast the fat on a fairly low heat –120–130°C (250–270°F) – for 2–3 hours, depending on the size of the piece. Pour the fat through cheese-cloth or a fine metal sieve. Store in glass jars and refrigerate.

Coconut oil is very good for cooking. It contains largely saturated fats and hence does not change its chemical structure when heated. Coconut oil contains anti-inflammatory and anti-microbial substances and is health giving. It has been used by traditional cultures for thou-sands of years and is one of the best fats to use for baking and cooking. Make sure that you buy natural coconut oil, which has not been hydrogenated, smoked or processed in any other way; it should smell and taste like fresh coconut. In cold temperatures it should be white and solid; in warm temperatures it will melt and become a slightly yellowish liquid.

SOUPS

Soups are a wonderful wholesome food, which balances your blood sugar level and reduces sugar cravings. Soups are quick and easy to make and, once made, a pot of soup will keep in the refrigerator for a few days, so you can always warm up a bowl for yourself. I strongly recommend making your soups with home-made meat stock. Meat stock aids digestion and has been known for centuries as a healing folk remedy, not only for the digestive tract, but also for many other organs of the body. Meat stock is extremely nourishing. It is full of minerals, vitamins, amino acids and various other nutrients in a very bio-avail-able form. Do not use commercially available stock granules or bouil-lon cubes; they are highly processed and full of detrimental ingredients.

Once you have made your meat stock, it can be frozen or will keep well in a refrigerator for at least a week. You can make soups, gravies and stews with the meat stock, or warm up a cup of it to have as a drink with meals or between meals. If you make sure that you always have some meat stock in your fridge, you will find that it is very easy and quick to make a warm nourishing meal for yourself and your family (please look at the basic soup recipe).

You need meat, joints and bones to make a good meat stock. Beef, lamb, pork, game, poultry and fish are all highly suitable and will make stocks with different flavours and different nutritional compositions. So, make sure that you alternate between different meats to provide a whole spectrum of nourishment. Bones and joints are particularly important as they enrich the stock with the kind of nourishing substances that meat alone cannot provide. In fact it can be very inexpensive to make a good-quality meat stock as you use the parts of the animal that butchers usually give away almost free. The meat and bones can be fresh or frozen and there is no need to defrost them prior to cooking. Apart from bones and meat, all you need is a large pot full of water and a bit of salt and pepper.

How to make meat stock

Lamb, pork, beef or game
Put the joints, bones and meat into a large pot, add 5–10 peppercorns (slightly crushed) and salt to taste. Fill with water. Heat up to boiling point. Cover the pan, reduce the heat to a minimum and simmer for 2–3 hours. The longer you cook the meat and bones, the more they will "give out" to the stock and the more nourishing the stock will be. Take the bones and meat out and pour the stock through a sieve into a separate pan to remove any small bones and peppercorns. Drinking this meat stock on a regular basis is one of the best remedies for arthritis and osteoporosis, as it provides collagen, gelatine and other nutrients essential for building bones and joints.

Chicken stock
Put a whole or half an organic chicken into a large pot, fill with water, add salt and heat to boiling point. Then reduce the heat to a minimum and simmer for 1½–2 hours. Take the chicken out and put the stock through a sieve. Keep in the refrigerator. The chicken, cooked this way, is delicious and can be served for dinner with vegetables and a hot cup of your freshly made chicken stock. This recipe is a must every time you, or your child, get a cold, a tummy bug, food poisoning or any other viral problem. Chicken stock is the best healing remedy in those situations: drink it hot all day, make a vegetable soup with it and eat it with the chicken (which you used for making the stock). Add 1–2

tablespoons of kefir or yoghurt into every bowl of soup. Do not eat anything else and your problem will soon be gone.

Fish stock

To make a good fish stock you need the bones, fins, skins and heads of fish, not the meat. So buy your fish whole, cut the meat off to cook as a separate meal and use the rest of the fish to make your stock. Your fishmonger can do all the trimming for you. Put the heads, bones, fins and skin into a large pan, add 8–10 peppercorns and fill the pan with water. Bring up to the boil, reduce the heat to a minimum and simmer for 1–1½ hours. Add salt to taste at the end of cooking. Take the fish out and sieve the stock. Take the meat off the fish skeleton to use for soup making.

Basic soup recipe

To make a soup bring some of your home-made meat stock to the boil, add chopped or sliced vegetables and simmer for another 20–25 minutes. You can choose any combination of available vegetables: onions, cabbages, carrots, broccoli, cauliflower, pumpkin, courgettes, marrow, squash, leeks, etc. If you are planning to blend your soup, you can cut vegetables roughly into any size pieces. If you prefer not to blend your soup, make sure that you cut or dice your vegetables into nice small pieces before cooking. If your meat stock was made with lamb, pork or beef, you can add a handful of dried French or Italian mushrooms for a wonderful flavour. It is customary to crush the dried mushrooms by hand before adding them to the soup. At the end of cooking, add 1–2 tablespoons of chopped garlic, bring to the boil and turn the heat off. Blend with a soup blender until smooth, unless you prefer it unblended.

You can serve your soup with any combination of the following:

- some chopped fresh parsley, coriander or dill
- hard-boiled egg cut into pieces
- a spoonful of yoghurt, kefir or crème fraiche
- cooked meat, cut into small pieces
- red onion, cut into very small pieces

- spring onion, cut into small pieces
- a spoonful of cooked and ground liver
- sunflower, sesame and pumpkin seeds (best sprouted)

If you have no time to make the soup, you can simply warm up a cup of your home-made meat stock and add any of the above to the cup to make a quick and nourishing meal for yourself.

From this basic recipe you can improvise and develop your own recipes. Here are just a few ideas.

Spring nettle soup

1½ litres home-made meat stock
large bunch of spring nettles
2 tablespoons dried French or Italian mushrooms
1 medium onion
1 medium carrot
2 courgettes or ¼ marrow or squash
4 eggs, hard boiled

The young shoots of stinging nettles that appear in spring are full of wonderful nourishment. They are high in iron, magnesium, copper, zinc, vitamin C, carotenoids and other useful substances. For this recipe, collect a large bunch of spring nettles. Wear gloves and a long-sleeved shirt when collecting the nettles. Rinse the nettles and shake off the excess water. Use scissors to cut the leaves and tender shoots into small pieces, discarding the hard stems. Reserve for the recipe.

Cut the marrow, squash or courgettes into small cubes, thinly slice the carrot and chop the onion. Bring some of your home-made meat stock to a boil. Add all the vegetables and the dried French or Italian mushrooms, crumbling them with your hands before adding to the meat stock. Simmer under a tight lid for 15–20 minutes. Add your prepared nettles, mix and immediately take off the heat. Serve with 1–2 tablespoons of hard-boiled egg, cut into small pieces, and a spoonful of yoghurt, kefir or crème fraiche.

Russian Borsch

1½ litres home-made meat stock
1 medium onion, finely chopped
1 medium carrot, finely sliced
¼ medium-size white cabbage, finely sliced
2 medium-size beetroots, or 4 small beetroots, raw or cooked
3 cloves garlic
1 tomato finely chopped

If the beetroot is cooked (in water, not in vinegar):
Bring the meat stock to the boil and add the onion, carrot and cabbage.
Cover and simmer for 20 minutes. In the meantime, slice the cooked
beetroots into long thin strips. Add to the soup, mix well and simmer
for another 5 minutes. Take off the heat. Crush the garlic and add to
the soup, together with the chopped tomato. Serve with a large spoonful of crème fraiche, kefir or yoghurt and some chopped parsley and/or
a thick slice of hard-boiled egg.

If the beetroot is raw:
Wash and peel the beetroot. Slice into long thin strips by hand or
using your food processor. Bring the meat stock to the boil and add the
beetroot. Simmer for 10–15 minutes, then add the rest of the vegetables (onion, carrot and cabbage). Simmer for a further 20 minutes or
until the cabbage is cooked. Take off the heat. Crush the garlic and add
to the soup, together with the chopped tomato. Serve with a large
spoon of crème fraiche or home-made yoghurt, some chopped parsley
and/or sliced hard-boiled egg.

Fish soup

1 litre home-made fish stock
large onion, finely chopped
1 carrot, thinly sliced
1 courgette, or equivalent amount of marrow or squash, cut into
small cubes

Bring the fish stock to the boil and add the onion, carrot and squash, marrow or courgettes. Simmer under a lid for 10–15 minutes and take off the heat. Add the cooked fish meat (which you took off the bones when you made the fish stock). Serve with a spoonful of fresh yoghurt or kefir and/or with a hard-boiled egg (sliced or chopped).

If there is no meat left on the bones you can use the meat (skinless and boneless) of any available fresh raw fish: just cut the meat into small cubes and add to the boiling fish stock at the same time as the vegetables.

Meatball soup

400g minced meat (a mixture of pork and beef is best)
1 large onion, finely chopped
1 large carrot, thinly sliced
1 cup winter squash or courgette, cut into small cubes
1 cup cabbage, finely chopped (optional)
2 tablespoons garlic, chopped
salt and cayenne pepper
2–3 tablespoons sauerkraut

In a pan bring 2 litres of water or meat stock (beef, pork or lamb) up to the boil. Add salt and cayenne pepper to taste.

With your hands shape the minced meat into balls about 2cm in diameter, and add them, one at a time, to the boiling water. Cover and simmer on low heat for 30 minutes. Add all the vegetables, apart from garlic, cover and simmer for another 20 minutes. Add the garlic and switch the heat off. Let the pan sit for 5–10 minutes to cool slightly, then add 2–3 tablespoons of sauerkraut. Serve with a spoonful of yoghurt, kefir or crème fraiche and finely chopped dill.

Beautiful winter squash soup

1½ litres home-made meat stock (turkey or chicken stock work
best for this recipe)
1 leek, washed and sliced
3–4 medium sized florets broccoli
1 medium-size carrot, sliced
½ medium-size buttercup squash, or ⅓ butternut squash or any
winter squash with sweet orange flesh
3 garlic cloves, peeled
double cream or crème fraiche

Peel and deseed the squash and cut it into chunks. Wash all the vegetables and cut into pieces. Put them in your soup pan, add the meat stock and bring to the boil. Reduce the heat to a minimum, cover with the lid and simmer for about 30 minutes. Blend with a soup blender, adding ½ cup of fresh double cream or crème fraiche to the soup. Serve warm.

Meat jelly (brawn)

2–4 pig trotters (the feet of the pig)
1 large carrot
garlic
salt
1–2 teaspoons black peppercorns

Put pig trotters into a large pan, fill it with water, add salt and black peppercorns (slightly crushed). Bring to the boil, then reduce the heat to a minimum, cover with a lid and simmer for 3 hours.

In the meantime, steam a large carrot until a knife goes through easily, cool and cut into thin slices. You can cut it into decorative slices if you have the right tools.

When the meat stock is ready, take the pig trotters out and pour the stock through a sieve into a separate pan. Let the trotters cool down completely. Take all the meats (including the skin and other soft tissues) from the trotters, completely stripping the bones. Cut the meat into small pieces.

In a large deep tray, lay the pieces of meat, the carrot slices and thin slices of garlic. You can add more or less garlic, to your family's taste. Pour in the meat stock until the tray is ¾ full. Place it in the refrigerator for the jelly to set. You can also set this jelly in different jelly shapes and dishes as individual servings.

This dish is wonderful on a hot summer's day. It contains a lot of nourishing substances, including gelatine, glucosamine, glycoproteins, phospholipids and others, and is a folk remedy for digestive problems, arthritis and osteoporosis.

SALADS

To increase the nutritional value of your salads it is good to sprinkle coarsely chopped walnuts or seeds on top. Seeds – sunflower, pumpkin and sesame – should be soaked in water overnight. It makes them more nourishing and easier to digest. If you do not use all the soaked seeds, just cover them with a damp cloth and let them sprout, which will make them even more nourishing.

Beetroot salad

8 small beetroots
½ cup shelled walnuts
2 cloves garlic
8 dried prunes without stones
mayonnaise
teaspoon salt

Wash the beetroots and cut off all tops and ends. Steam the beetroot until a knife goes through easily. Alternatively, you can buy cooked beetroots (in water, not vinegar!). Grate the beetroot with a coarse grater. In a food processor chop together walnuts, garlic and prunes. Mix well with the grated beetroot. Add salt and mayonnaise and mix. Enjoy with meats and vegetables.

Tuna salad

200g canned tuna in its own juice or water
1 large onion
2 large carrots
2 hard-boiled eggs
mayonnaise

Drain the tuna and mash with a fork. Chop the onion finely. Cook the carrots. Peel and chop the hard-boiled eggs.

On a flat dish put a layer of tuna (use half the tuna) and top with half the chopped onion. Cover with mayonnaise. Grate one carrot on top and cover with mayonnaise. Make a layer of one chopped hard-boiled egg and cover with mayonnaise. Repeat the same layers of tuna, onion, carrot and egg. Decorate with some dill or parsley. Make sure that every layer is well covered with mayonnaise.

Salad with cabbage and apple

100g white cabbage
1 large apple
½ cup home-made yoghurt or crème fraiche
1 teaspoon honey
pinch salt
2 tablespoons raisins

Grate the cabbage. Peel, core and grate the apple. Slightly fry the raisins in butter to soften them. Mix honey and salt with yoghurt. Mix all ingredients together.

Salad with tomatoes and cucumber

2 tomatoes
¹/₃ long cucumber
1 stick celery
spring onion
dill or parsley
salt

Cut cucumber into ½ cm slices. Cut tomato into bite-size pieces and slice the celery into small pieces. Sprinkle with salt. Chop the spring onions, dill and parsley. Mix all ingredients and dress with cold-pressed olive oil.

Russian salad

½ long cucumber
1 large carrot, cooked (steamed)
100g cooked meat or sausages (leftovers are good)
1 onion
2 hard-boiled eggs
2 tablespoons sauerkraut (optional)
fresh dill and/or parsley
⅓ teaspoon salt
mayonnaise
yoghurt or crème fraiche

Cut cucumber and carrot into small cubes. Cut the meat and/or sausages into small pieces. Finely chop the onion. Cut the eggs into small cubes. Finely chop dill and parsley. In a separate pot mix mayonnaise and yoghurt in equal proportions and add salt. Mix all ingredients together.

Carrot salad

1 large carrot
1 tablespoon raisins
1 tablespoon walnuts, coarsely chopped
yoghurt

Slightly fry the raisins in butter to soften them. Finely grate the carrot. Mix the carrot, raisins, walnuts and yoghurt.

MAIN DISHES

Italian meat casserole

This is an alternative way of making an excellent meat stock, as well as preparing a meal for the whole family. You can use any of the following: a leg or a shoulder of lamb, a joint of pork, a joint of beef, a pheasant, 2–4 pigeons, 2 quails, a joint of venison, a whole chicken, turkey legs. You need a large casserole with a lid. Put your meat joint or whole bird(s) into the casserole, add water to fill   of the casserole, add salt, peppercorns, dried herbs to taste, sun-dried tomatoes, bay leaves and a sprig of rosemary. Cover and place in the oven for 5–6 hours on low heat 125–140°C (250°F). About 40–50 minutes before your dinner time add various vegetables to the casserole: florets of broccoli and cauliflower, small peeled red or white onions, Brussels sprouts and large pieces of carrot. When ready take the meat and vegetables out and serve to your family. Put the meat stock through a sieve and serve it in bouillon cups with the dinner. Leftover meat stock will keep well in the refrigerator and can be used for making soups or as a warm nourishing drink.

Stuffed peppers

6 large peppers (a combination of green, red, yellow and orange)
½ kg minced meat (a mixture of ½ pork and ½ beef is best)
2 medium-size carrots
1 large onion
salt and pepper

Grate the carrots and chop the onion. Mix well with the minced meat, adding salt and pepper to taste.

   Cut off the tops of the peppers and remove the seeds. Fill the peppers with the meat and vegetables mixture. Place the stuffed peppers upright in a pan. You will need the correct size pan to fit all the peppers, so they stand upright and support each other. Add 3–4 cups of water to the bottom of the pan and cover. Bring up to the boil, reduce the heat to a minimum and simmer for an hour. Serve 1–2 peppers per person with a ladle of the stock from the bottom (best served in a soup bowl). On top of the pepper put a tablespoon of live yoghurt with a clove of crushed garlic mixed into it. Garnish with chopped parsley.

Meatballs

500g minced meat (a mixture of pork and beef is best)
1 large onion
½ red pepper
1 courgette
2 tablespoons fresh garlic, chopped
1 tablespoon tomato puree
salt and pepper
2–3 bay leaves
coriander

To make the sauce cover the bottom of a pan with 3–4 cm of water. Mix in tomato puree, salt and pepper. Bring to the boil. With your hands shape the minced meat into balls about 4cm in diameter. Put the balls one at a time in the boiling sauce. Make sure that you use a large enough pan to fit all the balls in one layer. Cover and simmer on low heat for 30 minutes.

In the meantime, prepare the vegetables. Finely chop the onion and red pepper. Cut the courgette into small cubes. Chop the garlic.

After cooking the meatballs for 30 minutes, add the chopped onion, pepper and courgette. Mix gently with the sauce preserving the shape of the meatballs. Cover and cook for another 25 minutes. Add the bay leaves and garlic. Cover and turn the heat off. Let the pan sit for 10 minutes before serving. Sprinkle with finely chopped coriander and serve with cooked vegetables and a fresh salad.

Meat cutlets

500g minced pork
500g minced beef or lamb
1 large onion, finely chopped
salt and pepper to taste

Mix all the ingredients well and make oval-shaped cutlets. In a frying pan warm up some pork dripping (goose or duck fat) and fry the cutlets slightly on both sides. Place the cutlets in a greased baking tray, add ½ cup of water and bake in the oven for 40 minutes at 150–170°C (300–350°F). Serve with cooked vegetables and a fresh salad.

Fish cutlets

2–3 fairly large freshwater or sea fish (a mixture of different fish works very well)
1 egg
3–5 tablespoons butter (ghee, goose fat, duck fat, pork dripping or coconut oil)
1–2 cups shredded coconut
salt and pepper

Cut all the meat off the fish, remove skin and large bones. Use the bones, heads and skin for making a very nourishing fish stock (recipe in the *soup* section). Alternatively you can buy fish fillets, already without skin and large bones.

In the food processor put the meat of the fish, egg, butter, salt and pepper to your taste, and grind it to make mince. If you have a meat mincer it will do the same job for you. With your hands make oval-shaped flat cutlets, about 2cm thick, roll them in shredded coconut and slightly fry them on both sides. Use coconut oil (butter, ghee, pork dripping, lard, goose fat or duck fat) for frying. Transfer the cutlets to a large oven tray, greased with any of the listed fats. Add ½ cup water and place in a preheated oven. Bake for 20–30 minutes at 150°C (300°F).

Marinated wild salmon

Good-quality salmon, such as fresh wild salmon, is best eaten uncooked. This way you will get all the best nutrients from the fish, including very valuable omega-3 fats. Raw fish is much easier to digest than cooked fish, and marinating removes any danger of infection or parasites. You need fresh wild salmon for this recipe.

6 boneless wild salmon fillets with skins on
3–4 large fresh lemons
1 teaspoon salt
1 teaspoon grainy mustard
2 teaspoons finely chopped fresh dill or ½ teaspoon dill seeds
½ teaspoon coarsely ground black pepper

To make the marinade: cut lemons in half and squeeze out all the juice,
use a knife to scoop all the flesh out of the lemons. Mix in salt, pepper,
mustard and dill.

Wash the fish. Find a glass dish that will just fit three fillets. Lay
three fillets of fish close together, skins down. Pour the marinade over
them and lay the other three fillets on top, skins up. Press down well
and lay a heavy weight on top of the fish, so the marinade almost
covers it. The fish needs to be submerged in the marinade, because if
any of it is left dry it may spoil. If any parts of the fish are not covered
by marinade, just add a little bit of water or more lemon juice.

Cover with a towel and leave in the refrigerator to marinade for 24
hours.

When ready, peel the skin off the fish (it comes off very easily) and
cut the fish into bite-size pieces. Serve with avocado and drizzle lemon
juice over it.

Swedish gravlax

skinless and boneless salmon fillet (it must be very fresh)
1 litre water at room temperature
1½ tablespoons salt
1 tablespoon honey
fresh dill
coarsely ground black pepper

Cut the fish into 0.5cm slices and place in a dip tray (any baking tray
will do). Sprinkle with finely chopped dill and black pepper. Dissolve
the salt and the honey in the water to make brine. Cover the fish with
the brine and leave at room temperature for 1–1½ hours. Pour off the
water and serve the fish with lettuce and mayonnaise.

This dish works particularly well with wild salmon. Because the fish is not cooked all the essential fatty acids and other nutrients are preserved. Refrigerate and consume within two days.

Baked beans or French cassoulet

Commercially available baked beans are full of sugar and are best avoided. This recipe will allow you to enjoy baked beans at home. Once you have made this dish, it will keep for a long time in the fridge or you can freeze it.

500g white (navy) beans
1 duck
1 tablespoon cider vinegar
1 teaspoon sea salt
2 tablespoons tomato puree
cayenne pepper
black pepper
5–6 bay leaves
sprig rosemary
1 teaspoon thyme

Soak the beans in water for 12–24 hours, drain, rinse well in cold water and drain again. Soaking and rinsing removes harmful substances from the beans.

Cut all the meat from the duck – the legs, wings, breasts – and all the fat. Cut the meat into chunks and the fat into small pieces. You can use the carcase of the duck and the giblets for making meat stock later. In a large pan put 2 litres of water, cider vinegar, sea salt, tomato puree, a pinch each of cayenne pepper and black pepper, bay leaves, rosemary and thyme. Mix in the beans and the duck pieces (the meat and the fat). Cover the pan with a lid and place in the oven. Cook at 120°C (250°F) for 4–5 hours. Check occasionally. If the beans are getting dry, add more water.

Serve hot. The baked beans left from this meal will keep in the fridge for a long time and can be served with other dishes.

Liver pudding

100g liver (calf or lamb)
1 egg
2 tablespoons butter (ghee, goose/duck fat)
1 medium-size onion
salt
parsley

Soak the liver in milk for a few hours to remove any bitter taste (optional). Wash the liver, dry with a paper towel and blend into a pulp in the food processor. Put through a sieve to remove any hard bits. Add salt, egg yolk, butter, finely chopped parsley and finely chopped onion. Whip the egg white stiff and fold into the mixture. Put the mixture in a suitable dish, cover with a sheet of baking paper and cook with steam. You can use a steamer or a large pan. To steam in a pan put some water at the bottom of the pan and place the dish in it. Make sure that you do not have too much water in the pan, as it will get into the dish with the liver. Cover the pan with a lid and place on the stove. Steam for about 1 hour. Serve with cooked vegetables and a salad.

Lamb's liver and hearts in a clay pot

100g liver (calf or lamb)
100g lamb's hearts
1 large onion
10 dried prunes with stones
1 large pot double cream, natural yoghurt or soured cream (you can use your home-made yoghurt or replace with ½ cup butter/ ghee)
a pinch of allspice
salt and pepper

Soak the liver in milk for a few hours to remove any bitter taste (optional). Wash and dry the liver and cut into small pieces with scissors. Cut the lamb's hearts into small pieces using scissors. In a suitable-size clay pot put the liver and lamb's hearts, finely chopped onion and prunes. Mix the cream (or yoghurt or sour cream) with salt, pepper and allspice, and add to the clay pot. Mix with the meats. Cover the pot with the lid or foil. Bake in the oven for about 1 hour at 160°C (320°F).

Quick liver recipe

100g liver
1 large onion
6–7 cloves of garlic
½ cup butter/ghee (goose/duck fat)
fresh parsley or dill

Soak the liver in milk for a few hours to remove any bitter taste (optional). Wash and dry the liver and cut into small pieces using scissors. In a frying pan melt the butter/ghee, add the sliced onion and finely chopped garlic. Fry slightly until the onion and garlic start turning golden. Add the liver, salt and pepper and stir-fry for about 4–5 minutes. Sprinkle chopped parsley or dill on top and drizzle with olive oil. Serve immediately.

Baked vegetables

You can bake any combination of the following vegetables:

onions, (white or red or shallots)
peppers (red, yellow, orange or green)
Brussels sprouts
courgettes or marrow
pumpkin
winter squashes
large mushrooms
turnips
aubergines (eggplant)
duck or goose fat

Peel the onion and cut into halves or quarters. Shallots do not need to be peeled, just bake them in their skins.

Cut the peppers into quarters, remove seeds.

Peel the outer leaves from Brussels sprouts.

Peel and cut into large chunks the courgettes, marrow and pumpkin. Remove the seeds from the pumpkin and the marrow. Rub the courgettes and marrow with salt.

Peel and slice the winter squash and remove the seeds.

Peel the turnips and cut like potato chips.

Cut the aubergine into chunks and rub with salt.

Rub plenty (a large handful at least) of goose or duck fat on the vegetables, place them on a baking tray and bake at 150°C (300°F) for 20–40 minutes, or until a sharp knife goes through easily. Serve with meat or fish.

BAKING AT HOME

Basic bread/cake/muffin recipe

2½ cups ground almonds
¼ cup softened butter (coconut oil, goose fat, duck fat or home-made yoghurt or crème fraiche)
3 eggs

You can buy ground almonds in most health-food shops. Instead of ground almonds you can use walnuts, pecans, hazelnuts, almonds, sunflower and pumpkin seeds, peanuts, cashew nuts, pine nuts and any combination of these. Grind them in your food processor to a flour consistency.

Mix all the ingredients well. You may want to add more or less ground almonds to reach porridge-like consistency. Grease your baking pan with butter or ghee, line it with greased baking paper and add the mixture to it. Bake in the oven at 150°C (300°F) for about an hour. Check occasionally with a dry, clean knife. If the knife comes out dry, then the bread is ready.

This is your basic recipe.

To make variations of this bread you can add some salt, pepper, dried herbs, tomato puree, sun-dried tomatoes, peanut butter, grated cheese (mature cheddar, parmesan or any other hard, full-bodied cheese), nuts, seeds, dried fruit, fresh or frozen berries, chunks of cooking apple, grated carrot, chunks of pumpkin (without the skin and seeds).

If you want to sweeten the mixture add 1½ cups dried fruit (dates, apricots, raisins, figs) or 2 ripe bananas. If the dried fruit is too hard, soak it in water for a few hours to soften or gently bring to boil with some water. You can also use ½ cup honey to sweeten the mixture. However, honey tends to burn and make your cake very brown. It is best to use dried fruit.

If you want the mixture to be softer and more moist, replace 1 cup ground almonds with any of the following: fresh pumpkin, butternut squash, any winter squash or courgettes. Peel and remove the seeds, blend into a pulp in your food processor and mix with the rest of the ingredients. You can also use carrot pulp from your juicer.

Improvise by trying your own variations. You can bake this mixture as a bread or cake, or in small paper cups as muffins, or make a pizza base. If you add more eggs and less ground almonds you can make pancakes and waffles. It really is very easy and manageable, even for the most inexperienced cook. These kinds of breads, muffins, waffles and pancakes will keep your blood sugar at a healthy level, provide you with lots of magnesium, amino acids and many other wonderful nutrients – and they taste divine!

DESSERTS

Baked apples

With a sharp knife scoop out the cores and seeds from large cooking apples. Fill each apple with a teaspoon of honey, a teaspoon of butter, ground or coarsely chopped apricot kernels (or walnuts, any other available nuts, or desiccated coconut). Add a dried apricot per apple (optional), cut into small pieces. Bake in the oven at 160–180°C (320–360°F) for 20–25 minutes.

Crème caramel

For one person you need:
1 egg
3 tablespoons water or milk
1 teaspoon honey
ground cinnamon

Multiply the ingredients per number of people you want to serve.
Mix all the ingredients well. Pour into shallow ramekin dishes (or any
other small terracotta dishes). You need one ramekin dish per person.
Sprinkle some cinnamon on top. Preheat the oven to 150°C (300°F).
Bake for 30–40 minutes.

Apple crumble

4 cooking apples
4 eggs
carrot pulp from juicing 2lb carrots, or 1lb carrots, finely grated
10 dried apricots
1 cup roughly chopped walnuts
½ cup honey
½ cup unsalted butter

Core and peel the apples, cut into pieces and place on the bottom of
your baking dish. Chop apricots into small pieces.
    Mix together eggs, walnuts, butter, carrot pulp, chopped apricots
and honey. Put the mixture on top of the apples, mixing slightly with
the apples. Bake in the oven at 150°C (300°F) for approximately 40
minutes.

Apple pie

4 large cooking apples
a handful of raisins
½ cup honey
1 cup fresh or frozen blackcurrants
2–3 cups fresh pumpkin, peeled and finely chopped
2 cups pitted dried dates
1 cup hazelnuts
½ cup ground almonds

Soak the dates in 2 cups of water for 2–3 hours. Drain the dates and reserve. Pour the soaking water into your baking dish. Add cored and sliced apples, raisins and blackcurrants. Spread them evenly and sprinkle with the ground almonds. Pour honey on top, spreading evenly.

In a food processor blend the dates, pumpkin and hazelnuts. Spoon this mixture on top of the pie, spreading evenly. Slightly press and smooth with a spoon or a knife so that the top looks like the top of a pie. Bake at 150–170°C (300–350°F) for an hour.

Winter squash cake

6 eggs
2 cups peeled and grated (packed tightly) winter squash with sweet orange flesh (buttercup, butternut or other)
½ cup honey
cup butter (ghee, coconut fat, goose fat or duck fat)
3 cups ground almonds
3 medium-size apples

Grease your baking dish and cover the bottom with apples, cored and cut into slices.

Blend the rest of the ingredients in your blender and put the mixture on top of the apples. Smooth the top and bake at 150°C (300°F) for 40–50 minutes.

Cake Pinocchio

2 cups shelled hazelnuts
1 cup honey (250ml)
4 eggs
50g unsalted butter, preferably organic
4 tangerines to decorate

Preheat the oven to 175–200°C (350–400°F).

Roast the hazelnuts in the oven and rub off their skins. Reserve 1 cup of the nuts for the cream and grind the rest into coarse flour.

Cut 4 circles out of baking paper to fit your cake dish and grease them with butter.

Separate the whites of the eggs from the yolks. Whip the egg whites stiff with half of the honey. Carefully fold in the ground hazelnuts. Spread the mixture on the four baking paper circles; place them on your baking tray and bake for 5–10 minutes. Cool down and remove the baking paper.

Cream Soften the butter by leaving it in the room for a few hours. Whip the egg yolks with the rest of the honey until they increase in volume and become pale in colour. Beat in the butter gradually, adding it in small amounts.

Coarsely chop the rest of the hazelnuts, reserving 10–15 whole nuts for decorating.

In your cake dish layer the meringue circles with the cream, sprinkling every cream layer with the coarsely chopped hazelnuts. Cover the top with a thin layer of the cream. Peal the tangerines and separate them into segments. Decorate the top with the segments and the 10–15 whole hazelnuts. Refrigerate.

Peanut butter pie

6 eggs
2 tablespoons butter
1 cup peanut butter
2 cups carrot pulp left after juicing carrots (you can use winter squash as a substitute, peel it and chop very finely)
½ cup honey
1 cup ground almonds
2 large cooking apples
a handful of raisins

Peel and core the apples, cut them into small pieces and place them into a greased baking dish. Sprinkle the raisins on top of the apples.

In a blender put the rest of the ingredients and blend well. Place the mixture on top of the apples. Smooth the top and bake at 150°C (300°F) for 40–50 minutes.

Russian custard

for one person:
2 egg yolks
½–1 teaspoon honey
multiply the ingredients for the number of people to be served

Russian custard can be used instead of cream on fruit, or you can serve it on its own with some chopped nuts or pieces of fruit on the top. It can also be used instead of cream in making cakes. Separate the egg yolks from the whites, add the honey and whip the mixture until it goes thick and almost white. As well as being a delicious desert, it provides very good nutrition. Get your eggs from a source you trust. Free-range, organic eggs are the best.

Apple sauce

5–6 large cooking apples
½ cup butter
1–2 cups water
2 cups honey

Peel and core the apples, cut them into pieces and cook in a pan with the water until soft. Take off the heat and add butter. Cool down, mash and sweeten with honey.

You can make pear sauce the same way, though you may not need to add honey, as pears are naturally very sweet.

This sauce will keep well in the refrigerator and can be served with some yoghurt, double cream, chopped nuts, Russian custard or on its own.

Birthday cake

6 eggs
2 cups ground almonds
550ml fresh double cream
2 cups honey
1 kg fresh or frozen raspberries
1 large bar good-quality dark chocolate
colourful fruit to decorate

Separate the yolks and whites of the eggs into two large bowls. Whip the yolks until thick and light in colour. Whip the whites until firm and no longer runny. Add some of the whites to the yolks and mix gently, then add the ground almonds to that mixture. Mix well (you can use a food processor), then gradually fold in the whites mixing gently with a spoon (not with a food processor). Bake in a cake tin lined with greased baking paper for 40–60 minutes at a temperature of 150°C (300°F). Test with a dry knife (the knife will come out dry if the cake is ready). Depending on the oven, the baking time may vary. When ready allow the cake to cool down.

Combine the cream and honey and whip until stiff.

Now the fun part starts. With a long knife cut off the top of the cake making sure that this layer is no more than 1cm thick. Put it aside for later. Using a tablespoon, carefully spoon out the inside of the cake in medium-sized chunks and place them in a separate dish, leaving just an outside shell, which will look like a dish ready to be filled. Fill it up with layers of whipped cream, frozen raspberries and chunks of spooned-out cake. When the "cake dish" is filled, cover it with the top layer that you removed earlier. Spread the remaining cream on the sides and the top of the cake.

Break the chocolate bar into pieces, place them in a bowl, add 4–5 tablespoons of water and melt over hot steam, constantly mixing. Add more water if the chocolate is too thick. When the chocolate is fairly liquid, pour it over the whole cake. The cake is now ready to be decorated.

To decorate you can use fresh fruit, berries, nuts and desiccated coconut. When decorating is done, put the cake into the refrigerator. It is best to make this cake the day before the party so it has time to "mature" overnight.

References

Introduction

1. Coronary Heart Disease Statistics 2012; British Heart Foundation.
2. Nichols M, Townsend N, Scarborough P, et al; Cardiovascular disease in Europe: epidemiological update. *Eur Heart J.* 2013 Oct.
3. 34(39):3028–34. doi: 10.1093/eurheartj/eht356. Epub 2013 Sep 7.
4. Gaziano TA, et al. Growing Epidemic of Coronary Heart Disease in Low- and Middle-Income Countries. *Curr Probl Cardiol.* 2010 Feb; 35(2): 72–115. PMCID: PMC2864143.
5. Falk E. Pathogenesis of atherosclerosis. *J Am Coll Cardiol.* 2006; 47:7–12.
6. Guyton and Hall (2011). *Textbook of Medical Physiology.* U.S.: Saunders Elsevier.
7. Ravnskov U. *The Cholesterol Myths. Exposing the fallacy that saturated fat and cholesterol cause heart disease.* 2000. NewTrends Publishing.

Part One: The Myths

The diet-heart hypothesis

1. Keys A. Atherosclerosis: A problem in newer public health. *Journal of Mount Sinai Hospital* 20, 118–139, 1953.
2. Reiser RA. A commentary on the rationale of the diet-heart statement of the American Heart Association. *American Journal of Clinical Nutrition* 40, 654–658, 1984.
3. Mann GV. Coronary heart disease: "Doing the wrong things." *Nutrition Today* July/August, p.12–14, 1985.
4. Rosch PJ. Statins don't work by lowering lipids. *British Medical Journal* 2001, 17.
5. Rosch PJ. Views on Cholesterol. *Health and Stress. The Newsletter of The American Institute of Stress*, Volumes 1995: 1, 1998: 1, 1999: 8, 2001: 2,4,7.
6. Enig MG. *Know Your Fats: The Complete Primer for Understanding the Nutrition of Fats, Oils, and Cholesterol.* Bethesda Press, Silver Spring, MD, 2000.
7. Stehbens WE. The lipid hypothesis and the role of hemodynamics in atherogenesis. *Progress in Cardiovascular Diseases.* 33, 119–136, 1990.
8. Smith RL. Diet, blood cholesterol and coronary heart disease: a critical review of the literature. *Vector Enterprises.* Vol.1, 1989; Vol. 2, 1991.

9. Werko L. The enigma of coronary heart disease and its prevention. *Acta Medica Scandinavica* 221, 323–333, 1987.

10. Werko L. Analysis of the MRFIT screenees: a methodological study. *Journal of Internal Medicine* 237, 507–518, 1995.

11. Pinckney E, Pinckney C. *The Cholesterol Controversy.* Sherbourne Press. Los Angeles, 1973.

12. Ravnskov U. *The Cholesterol Myths. Exposing the fallacy that saturated fat and cholesterol cause heart disease.* 2000. NewTrends Publishing.

13. Mann GV, Shaffer RD, Rich A. Physical fitness and immunity to heart disease in Masai. *The Lancet* 2, 1308–1310, 1965.

14. Shaper AG. Cardiovascular studies in the Samburu tribe of northern Kenya. *American Heart Journal* 63, 437–442, 1962.

15. Kannel WB, Gordon T. The Framingham diet study: diet and the regulation of serum cholesterol. The Framingham study. An Epidemiological Investigation of Cardiovascular Disease. Section 24. Washington, DC, 1970.

16. Taubes G. Nutrition: The soft science of dietary fat. *Science magazine* 292, 2536–2545, 2001.

17. Marmot MG et al. Epidemiologic studies of coronary heart disease and stroke in Japanese men living in Japan, Hawaii and California: Prevalence of coronary and hypertensive heart disease and associated risk factors. *American Journal of Epidemiology* 102, 514–525, 1975.

18. Oliver MF. Doubts about preventing coronary heart disease. Multiple interventions in middle-aged men may do more harm than good. *British Medical Journal* 304, 393–394, 1992.

19. Texon M. *Hemodynamic basis for atherosclerosis with critique of the cholesterol-heart disease hypothesis.* Begell House, New York, 1995.

20. Green WH. *The Cholesterol Conspiracy.* Inc. St. Louis, 1991.

21. Gould KL. "Very low-fat diets for coronary heart disease: Perhaps, but which one?" *JAMA* 275: 1402–1403 (1996).

22. Weidman WH et al. Nutrient intake and serum cholesterol level in normal children 6 to16 years of age. *Pediatrics* 61, 354–359, 1978.

23. Atrens DM. The questionable wisdom of a low-fat diet and cholesterol reduction. *Social Science and Medicine* 39, 433–447, 1994.

24. Nichols AB et al. Daily nutritional intake and serum lipid levels. The Tecumseh study. *American Journal of Clinical Nutrition* 29, 1384–1392, 1976.

25. Morris JN et al. Diet and plasma cholesterol in 99 bank men. *British Medical Journal* 1, 571–576, 1963.

26. Marek Z et al. Atherosclerosis and levels of serum cholesterol in post-mortem investigations. *American Heart Journal* 63, 768–774, 1962.

27. Apfelbaum M. *Vivre avec du cholesterol.* Editions du Rocher, Monaco 1992.

28. Smith GD, Pekkanen J. Should there be a moratorium on the use of cholesterol lowering drugs? *British Medical Journal* 304, 431–434, 1992.

29. Berger M The cholesterol non-consensus. In: Somogyi JC, Biro G, Hotzel D (eds): *Nutrition and Cardiovascular Risks*. Bibliotheca Nutritio et Dieta nr 49, 125–130, 1992.

30. McGee CT. *Heart Frauds. Uncovering the Biggest Health Scam in History*. HealthWise, Colorado Springs, 2001.

31. Ravnskov U. High cholesterol may protect against infections and atherosclerosis. *Q J Med* 2003; 96: 927–34.

32. Ravnskov U, Rosch PJ, Langsjoen PH, Kauffman JM, McCully KS. Evidence from the simvastatin trials that cancer is a probable long-term side effect. Unpublished letter to *The Lancet*.

33. Rosch PJ. Statin Associated Peripheral Neuropathy. *Lancet*, in press.

34. Golomb BA, Kane T, Dimsdale JE. Severe irritability associated with statin cholesterol-lowering drugs. *Quart J M* 2004; 97: 229–235.

35. Golomb BA. Statin adverse effects. *Geriatric Times* 2004; 5.

36. Wagstaff LR, Mitton MW, Arvik BM, Doraiswamy PM. Statin-associated memory loss: analysis of 60 case reports and review of the literature. *Pharmacotherapy* 2003 Jul; 23(7): 871–80.

37. Edison RJ, Muenke M. Central nervous system and limb anomalies in case reports of first-trimester statin exposure. *N Engl J Med* 2004; 350: 1579–1582.

38. Kendrick M. We are sleep-walking into what could become a major medical disaster because statin drugs will soon be sold over-the-counter. *Red Flags Daily,* June 17, 2004.

39. Rundek T, Naini A, Sacco R, Coates K, DiMauro S. Atorvastatin decreases the coenzyme Q10 level in the blood of patients at risk for cardiovascular disease and stroke. *Arch Neurol.* 2004; 61: 889–92.

40. Dam H, Sondergaard E. The encephalomalacia – producing effect of arachidonic and linoleic acids. *Zeitschrift fur Ernahrungswissenschaft* 2, 217–222, 1962.

41. Richie J et al. Oedema and haemolytic anaemia in premature infants. *New England Journal of Medicine* 279, 1185–1190, 1968.

42. Pinckney ER. The potential toxicity of excessive polyunsaturates. Do not let the patient harm himself. *American Heart Journal* 85, 723–726, 1973.

43. West CE, Redgrave TG. Reservations on the use of polyunsaturated fats in human nutrition. *Search* 5, 90–96, 1974.

44. McHugh MI et al. Immunosuppression with polyunsaturated fatty acids in renal transplantation. *Transplantation* 24, 263–267, 1977.

45. Alexander JC, Valli VE, Chanin BE. Biological observations from feeding heated corn oil and heated peanut oil to rats. *Journal of Toxicology and Environmental Health* 21, 295–309, 1087.

46. Enig MG. Trans fatty acids in the food supply: a comprehensive report covering 60 years of research. Enig Associates, Inc., Silver Spring, MD, 1993.
47. Horrobin DF. Lowering cholesterol concentrations and mortality. *British Medical Journal* 301, 554, 1990.
48. Golomb BA. Cholesterol and violence: is there a connection? *Annals of Internal Medicine* 128, 478–487, 1998.
49. Koletzko B. Trans fatty acids may impair biosynthesis of long-chain polyunsaturates and growth in man. *Acta Pediatrica* 81, 302–306, 1992.
50. Gurr MI, James AT. *Lipid Biochemistry*. 3rd Edition, England, Chapman and Hall, 1980.
51. Stryer L. *Biochemistry*, 3rd Edition. New York, NY. W.H. Freeman & Co. 1988.
52. Mensick RP, Katan MB. Effect of dietary trans fatty acids on high-density and low-density lipoprotein cholesterol levels in healthy subjects. *New England Journal of Medicine* 323, 439–445, 1990.
53. Muldoon MF, Manuck SB, Matthews KA. Lowering cholesterol concentrations and mortality: a quantitative review of primary prevention trials. *British Medical Journal* 301, 554, 1990.
54. Lindberg G et al. Low serum cholesterol concentration and short term mortality from injuries in men and women. *British Medical Journal* 305, 277–279, 1992.
55. Editorial. Atherosclerosis and auto-oxidation of cholesterol. *The Lancet* 1, 964–965, 1980.
56. Steinberg D et al. Beyond cholesterol. Modification of low-density lipoprotein that increases its atherogenicity. *New England Journal of Medicine* 320, 915–924, 1989.
57. Iso H et al. Serum cholesterol levels and six-year mortality from stroke in 350,944 men screened for the multiple risk factor intervention trial. *New England Journal of Medicine* 320, 904–910, 1989.
58. Ravnskov U. Prevention of atherosclerosis in children. *The Lancet* 355, 69, 2000.
59. Castelli WP et al. Cardiovascular risk factors in the elderly. *American Journal of Cardiology* 63, 12H–19H, 1989.
60. Krumholz HM et al. Lack of association between cholesterol and coronary heart disease mortality and morbidity and all-cause mortality in persons older than 70 years. *Journal of the American Medical Association* 272, 1335–1340, 1994.
61. Shestov DB et al. Increased risk of coronary heart disease death in men with low total and low-density-lipoprotein cholesterol in the Russian Lipid Research Clinics; prevalence follow-up study. *Circulation* 99, 946–853,1993.

62. Forette B et al. Cholesterol as risk factor for mortality in elderly women. *The Lancet* 1, 868–870, 1989.
63. Frank GC, Berenson GS, Webber LS. Dietary studies and the relationship of diet to cardiovascular disease risk factor variables in 10-year-old children – the Bogalusa heart study. *The American Journal of Clinical Nutrition* 31, 328–340, 1978.
64. Tuomilehto J, Kuulasmaa K. WHO MONICA Project: Assessing CHD mortality and morbidity. *International Journal of Epidemiology* 18, suppl. 1, S38–S45, 1989.
65. Esrey KL et al. Relationship between dietary intake and coronary heart disease mortality: Lipid Research Clinics prevalence follow-up study. *Journal of Clinical Epidemiology* 49, 211–216, 1996.
66. Sherwin RW et al. Serum cholesterol levels and cancer mortality in 361,662 men screened for the multiple risk factor intervention trial. *Journal of the American Medical Association* 257, 943–948, 1987.
67. Cowan LD et al. Cancer mortality and lipid and lipoprotein levels. The Lipid Research Clinics' program mortality follow-up study. *American Journal of Epidemiology* 131, 468–482, 1990.
68. Buchwald H et al. Effect of partial ileal bypass surgery on mortality and morbidity from coronary heart disease in patients with hypercholesterolemia. Report of the program on the surgical control of the hyper lipidemias (POSCH). *New England Journal of Medicine* 323, 946–955, 1990.
69. Data from 1986 FAO Production Yearbook 40, 1987; and World Health Statistics Annual, 1993.
70. Dietschy JM, Turley SD. Cholesterol metabolism in the brain. *Curr Opin Lipidol*, 2001, 12: 105–112.
71. Jacobs D et al. Report of the conference on low blood cholesterol: Mortality associations. *Circulation* 86, 1046–1060, 1992.
72. Iribarren C et al. Serum total cholesterol and risk of hospitalisation and death from respiratory disease. *International Journal of Epidemiology* 26, 1191–1202, 1997.
73. Iribarren C et al. Cohort study of serum total cholesterol and in-hospital incidence of infectious diseases. *Epidemiology and Infection* 121, 335–347, 1998.
74. Claxton AJ et al. Association between serum total cholesterol and HIV infection in a high-risk cohort of young men. *Journal of Acquired Immune Deficiency Syndromes and Human Retrovirology* 17, 51–57, 1998.
75. Neaton JD, Wentworth DN. Low serum cholesterol and risk of death from AIDS. *AIDS* 11, 929–930, 1997.
76. Elias ER et al. Clinical effects of cholesterol supplementation in six patients with the Smith-Lemli-Opitz syndrome (SLOS). *American Journal of Medical Genetics* 68, 305–310, 1997.

77. Bhakdi S et al. Binding and partial inactivation of Staphylococcus aureus A-toxin by human plasma low density lipoprotein. *Journal of Biological Chemistry* 258, 5899–5904, 1983.
78. Muldoon MF et al. Immune system differences in men with hypo- or hypercholesterolemia. *Clinical Immunology and Immunopathology* 84, 145–149, 1997.
79. Graveline D. *Lipitor – thief of memory, statin drugs and the misguided war on cholesterol.* 2006. Infinity Publishing, Haverford, Pennsylvania.
80. Study suggests statins link to Parkinson's. *Natural Products*, Feb 2007, p. 6.
81. Graveline D. Statin Drugs Side Effects. 2008. www.spacedoc.net
82. Enig M. *Know Your Fats: The Complete Primer for Understanding the Nutrition of Fats, Oils and Cholesterol.* Silver Spring: Bethseda Press, 2000.

Part One: The Myths

Cholesterol: friend or foe?

1. Alberts et al. *Molecular Biology of the Cell*: 4th edition, NY: Garland Science, 2002.
2. Nelson DL and Cox MM. *Lehninger Principles of Biochemistry*, 4th edition, 2004.
3. Seeley RR, Stephens TD, Tate P. *Anatomy and physiology*, 2nd edition. Mosby Year Book, 1992.
4. Enig M. *Know Your Fats: The Complete Primer for Understanding the Nutrition of Fats, Oils and Cholesterol.* Silver Spring: Bethseda Press, 2000.
5. Garrow JS, James WPT, Ralph A. *Human nutrition and dietetics.* 10th edition. Churchill Livingstone, 2000.
6. Ravnskov U. *The Cholesterol Myths. Exposing the fallacy that saturated fat and cholesterol cause heart disease.* 2000. NewTrends Publishing.
7. Ravnskov U. Prevention of atherosclerosis in children. *The Lancet* 355, 69, 2000.
8. Strong JP, et al. Pathology and epidemiology of atherosclerosis. *J. Am. Diet. Assoc.* 62, 262–268 (1973).
9. Purves W, Sadava D, Orians G, and Heller C. 2004. *Life: The Science of Biology,* 7th edition. Sunderland, MA: Sinauer.
10. Berg JM, Tymoczko JL and Stryer L. *Biochemistry*, 2006.
11. Dietschy JM, Turley SD. Cholesterol metabolism in the brain. *Curr Opin Lipidol.* 2001, 12: 105–112.
12. Strauss E. Developmental Biology: one-eyed animals implicate cholesterol in development. *Science* 280; 1528–1529; 1998.

13. Sadler TW (1990). *Langman's medical embryology* (6th ed.). Williams and Wilkins.
14. Moore KL, Persaud TV. (2011). *The developing human – clinical oriented embryology*. 9th edition. USA: Saunders, an imprint of Elsevier Inc.
15. Huttenlocher PR, Dabholkar AS. (1997). "Regional differences in synaptogenesis in human cerebral cortex". *The Journal of Comparative Neurology* 387 (2).
16. Graveline D. *Lipitor – thief of memory, statin drugs and the misguided war on cholesterol*. 2006. Infinity Publishing, Haverford, Pennsylvania.
17. UCSF Medical Centre data: /ucsfhealth.org/education/cholesterol_content_of_foods
18. USDA food composition nutrient database online.
19. Graveline D. *The statin damage crisis*. 2014. Infinity Publishing.
20. Horrobin DF. Lowering cholesterol concentrations and mortality. *British Medical Journal* 301, 554, 1990.
21. Albert DJ et al. Aggression in humans: what is its biological foundation? *Neurosci Biobehav Rev.* 1993; 17: 405–425.
22. Muldoon MF, Manuck SB, Matthews KA. Lowering cholesterol concentrations and mortality: a quantitative review of primary prevention trials. *British Medical Journal* 301, 554, 1990.
23. Golomb BA. Cholesterol and violence: is there a connection? *Annals of Internal Medicine* 128, 478–487, 1998.
24. Bahrke MS et al. Psychological and behavioural effects of endogenous testosterone levels and anabolic-androgenic steroids among males. Review. *Sports Med.* 1990; 10: 303–337.
25. Bhasin S et al. Sexual dysfunction in men and women with endocrine disorders. *Lancet.* 2007 Feb 17; 369 (9561): 597–611. Review.
26. Chavarro JE et al. A prospective study of dairy foods intake and anovulatory infertility. *Human Reproduction*, issue 28, Feb 2007.
27. Hulley SB et al. Health policy on blood cholesterol. Time to change directions. *Circulation* 86, 1026–1029, 1992.
28. Guyton and Hall (2011). *Textbook of Medical Physiology*. U.S.: Saunders Elsevier.
29. Adams and Hollis. Vitamin D: synthesis, metabolism and clinical measurement. In: Coe and Favus, eds., *Disorders of Bone and Mineral Metabolism*, Philadelphia: Lippincott Williams and Wilkins (2002).
30. Jacobs D et al. Report of the conference on low blood cholesterol: 31. Mortality associations. *Circulation* 86, 1046–1060, 1992.
31. Rosch PJ. Views on Cholesterol. *Health and Stress. The Newsletter of The American Institute of Stress*, volumes 1995: 1, 1998: 1, 1999: 8, 2001: 2,4,7.
32. Skrabanek P, McCormick J. Follies and fallacies in medicine. Tarragon Press, Glasgow, 1989.

33. Elias ER et al. Clinical effects of cholesterol supplementation in six patients with the Smith-Lemli-Opitz syndrome (SLOS). *American Journal of Medical Genetics* 68, 305–310, 1997.
34. Leese HJ. What does an embryo need? *Hum Fertil (Camb)*. 2003 Nov; 6(4): 180–5. Review.
35. Luther JS et al. Nutritional paradigms of ovine foetal growth restriction: implications for human pregnancy. *Hum Fertil (Camb)*. 2005 Sep; 8(3): 179–87. Review.
36. Vitamin D: its role in cancer prevention and treatment. *Prog Biophys Mol Biol*. 2006 Sep; 92(1): 49–59. Epub 2006 Mar 10. Review.
37. Vitamin D physiology. *Prog Biophys Mol Biol*. 2006 Sep; 92(1): 4–8. Epub 2006 Feb 28. Review.
38. Vitamin D and cancer. *Anticancer Res*. 2006 Jul–Aug; 26(4A): 2515–24. Review.
39. Heaney RP. The vitamin D requirement in health and disease. *Journal of Steroid Biochemistry & Molecular Biology*, 97 (2005), 13–19.
40. An estimate of premature cancer mortality in the U.S. due to inadequate doses of solar ultraviolet-B radiation. *Cancer*. 2002 Mar 15; 94(6): 1867–75.
41. Beneficial effects of sun exposure on cancer mortality. *Prev Med*. 1993 Jan; 22(1): 132–40. Review.
42. Does sunlight prevent cancer? A systematic review. *Eur J Cancer*. 2006 Sep; 42(14): 2222–32. Epub 2006 Aug 10. Review.
43. Does sunlight have a beneficial influence on certain cancers? *Prog Biophys Mol Biol*. 2006 Sep; 92(1): 132–9. Epub 2006 Feb 28. Review.
44. Ecologic studies of solar UVB radiation and cancer mortality rates. Recent Results. *Cancer Res*. 2003; 164: 371–7. Review.
45. Geographic patterns of prostate cancer mortality. Evidence for a protective effect of ultraviolet radiation. *Cancer*. 1992 Dec 15; 70(12): 2861–9.
46. Multiple sclerosis and prostate cancer: what do their similar geographies suggest? *Neuroepidemiology*.1992; 11(4–6): 244–54.
47. Sunlight and vitamin D for bone health and prevention of autoimmune diseases, cancers, and cardiovascular disease. *Am J Clin Nutr*. 2004 Dec; 80(6 Suppl): 1678S–88S. Review.
48. UV radiation and cancer prevention: what is the evidence? *Anticancer Res*. 2006 Jul–Aug; 26(4A) :2723–7. Review.
49. Harris HW et al. The lipemia of sepsis: triglyceride-rich lipoproteins as agents of innate immunity. *Journal of Endotoxin Research* 6, 421–430, 2001.
50. Iribarren C et al. Serum total cholesterol and risk of hospitalisation and death from respiratory disease. *Int J Epidemiol* 26, 1191–1202, 1997.

51. Iribarren C et al. Cohort study of serum total cholesterol and in-hospital incidence of infectious diseases. *Epidemiology and Infection* 121, 335–347, 1998.
52. Bhakdi S et al. Binding and partial inactivation of Staphylococcus aureus A-toxin by human plasma low density lipoprotein. *Journal of Biological Chemistry* 258, 5899–5904, 1983.
53. Claxton AJ et al. Association between serum total cholesterol and HIV infection in a high-risk cohort of young men. *Journal of acquired immune deficiency syndromes and human retrovirology* 17, 51–57, 1998.
54. Muldoon MF et al. Immune system differences in men with hypo- or hypercholesterolemia. *Clinical Immunology and Immunopathology* 84, 145–149, 1997.
55. Neaton JD, Wentworth DN. Low serum cholesterol and risk of death from AIDS. *AIDS* 11, 929–930, 1997.
56. Ravnskov U. High cholesterol may protect against infections and atherosclerosis. *Q J Med* 2003; 96: 927–34.
57. Porter, Roy (2006). *The Cambridge History of Medicine*. Cambridge University Press.
58. Halliwell B, Gutteridge JMC. *Free radicals in biology and medicine.* Clarendon Press, Oxford 1989 (2nd ed.).
59. McMichael J. Fats and arterial disease. *American Heart Journal* 98, 409–412, 1979.
60. McGee CT. Heart Frauds. Uncovering the biggest health scam in history. HealthWise, Colorado Springs 2001.
61. Pfohl M, Schreiber I et al. Upregulation of cholesterol synthesis after acute myocardial infarction – is cholesterol a positive acute phase reactant? *Atherosclerosis,* Vol 142:2, Feb 1999, 389–393(5).
62. Elwood PC, Pickering JE and Fehily AM. Milk and dairy consumption, diabetes and the metabolic syndrome: the Caerphilly prospective study. *Journal of Epidemiology and Community Health* 2007; 61: 695–698.
63. Pizzorno JE, Murray MT. *Textbook of natural medicine.* 4th edition, 2012.
64. O'Brien JS, Sampson EL. Lipid composition of the normal human brain: gray matter, white matter and myelin. *Journal of Lipid Research,* Vol 6, 1965.

Part Two: What is Atherosclerosis?

Atherosclerosis is an inflammatory condition

1. Ross R. Atherosclerosis: an inflammatory disease. *N Engl J Med.* 1999; 340: 115–126.
2. Libby P, Ridker PM, Maseri A. Inflammation and atherosclerosis. *Circulation,* 2002; 105:1135.

3. Abou-Raya A, Abou-Raya S. Inflammation: a pivotal link between autoimmune diseases and atherosclerosis. *Autoimmun Rev.* 2006 May; 5(5): 331–7.
4. Danesh J, Whincup P, Walker M et al. Low grade inflammation and coronary heart disease: prospective study and updated meta-analyses. *BMJ.* 2000; 321: 199–204.
5. Nylaende M, Kroese A, Stranden E et al. Markers of vascular inflammation are associated with the extent of atherosclerosis assessed as angiographic score and treadmill walking distances in patients with peripheral arterial occlusive disease. *Vascular Medicine*, February 1, 2006; 11(1): 21–28.
6. Liuzzo G, Biasucci LM, Gallimore JR et al. The prognostic value of C-reactive protein and serum amyloid A protein in severe unstable angina. *N Engl J Med.* 1997; 331: 417–424.
7. Koenig W, Sung M, Frohlich M et al. C-reactive protein, a sensitive marker of inflammation, predicts future risk of coronary heart disease in initially healthy middle-aged men: results from the MONICA (Monitoring Trends and Determinants in Cardiovascular Disease) Augsburg Cohort Study, 1984 to 1992. *Circulation.* 1999; 99: 237–242.
8. Ridker PM, Hennekens CH, Buring JE et al. C-reactive protein and other markers of inflammation in the prediction of cardiovascular disease in women. *N Engl J Med.* 2000; 342: 836–843.
9. Ladwig KH, Marten-Mittag B, Lowel H et al. C-reactive protein, depressed mood, and the prediction of coronary heart disease in initially healthy men: results from the MONICA-KORA Augsburg Cohort Sturdy 1984–1998. *Eur. Heart J*, December 1, 2005; 26(23): 2537–2542.
10. Seeley RR, Stephens TD, Tate P. *Anatomy and physiology*, 2nd edition. Mosby Year Book, 1992.
11. Liuzzo G, Giubilato G, Pinnelli M. T cells and cytokines in atherogenesis. *Lupus*, September 1, 2005: 14(9): 732–735.
12. Zwaka TP, Hombach V, Torzewski J. C-reactive protein-mediated low density lipoprotein uptake by macrophages: implications for atherosclerosis. *Circulation.* 2001; 103; 1194–1197.
13. Torzewski M, Rist C, Mortensen RF et al. C-reactive protein in the arterial intima: role of C-reactive protein receptor-dependent monocyte recruitment in atherogenesis. *Arterioscler Thromb Vasc Biol.* 2000; 20: 2094–2099.
14. Hansson GK. Inflammation, atherosclerosis and coronary artery disease. *N Engl J Med* 2005; 352: 1685–1695.
15. Falk E. Pathogenesis of atherosclerosis. *J Am Coll Cardiol*, 2006; 47: 7–12.
16. Garrow JS, James WPT, Ralph A. *Human nutrition and dietetics*. 10th edition. Churchill Livingstone, 2000.

17. Warren H. Green. *The Cholesterol Conspiracy*. Inc. St. Louis, 1991.
18. Ravnskov U. High cholesterol may protect against infections and atherosclerosis. *Q J Med* 2003; 96: 927–34.
19. Pfohl M, Schreiber I et al. Upregulation of cholesterol synthesis after acute myocardial infarction – is cholesterol a positive acute phase reactant? *Atherosclerosis*, Vol 142:2, Feb 1999, 389–393(5).
20. Geng YJ, Libby P. Progression of atheroma, a struggle between death and procreation. *Arterioscler Thromb Vasc Biol* 2002; 22: 1370–1380.
21. Solberg LA, Strong JP. Risk factors and atherosclerotic lesions: a review of autopsy studies. *Arteriosclerosis*. 1983; 3: 187–198.
22. Kragel AH, Reddy SG, Wittes JT, Roberts WC. Morphometric analysis of the composition of atherosclerotic plaques in the four major epicardial coronary arteries in acute myocardial infarction and in sudden coronary death. *Circulation* 1989; 80: 1747–1756.
23. Enig MG. *Know Your Fats: The Complete Primer for Understanding the Nutrition of Fats, Oils, and Cholesterol*. 2000. Bethesda Press.
24. Willerson JT, Kereiakes DJ. Endothelial dysfunction. *Circulation* 2003; 108: 2060–2061.
25. Tousoulis D, Charakida M, Stefanadis C. Endothelial function and inflammation in coronary artery disease. *Heart*, April 1, 2006; 92(4): 441–444.
26. Virmani R, Kolodgie FD, Burke AP et al. Atherosclerotic plaque progression and vulnerability to rupture, angiogenesis as a source of intraplaque hemorrhage. *Arterioscler Thromb Vasc Biol* 2005; 25: 2054–2061.
27. Naruko T, Ueda M, Haze K et al. Neutrophil infiltration of culprit lesions in acute coronary syndromes. *Circulation* 2002; 106: 2894–2900.
28. Kaartinen M, Van Der Wal AC, Van Der Loos CM et al. Mast cell infiltration in acute coronary syndromes, implications for plaque rupture. *J Am Coll Cardiol* 1998; 32: 606–612.
29. Kilic T, Ural D, Ural E, Yumuk Z, Agacdiken A et al. Relation between proinflammatory to anti-inflammatory cytokine ratios and long-term prognosis in patients with non-ST elevation acute coronary syndrome. *Heart*, August 1, 2006; 92(8): 1041–1046.
30. Schwartz SM, Virmani R, Rosenfeld ME. The good smooth muscle cells in atherosclerosis. *Curr Atheroscler Rep* 2000; 2: 422–429.
31. Davies MJ, Woolf N, Rowles PM, Pepper J. Morphology of the endothelium over atherosclerotic plaques in human coronary arteries. *Br Heart J* 1988; 60: 459–464.
32. Vink A, Schoneveld AH, Richard W et al. Plaque burden, arterial remodelling, and plaque vulnerability determined by systemic factors? *J Am Coll Cardiol*. 2001;38:718–723.

33. Sata M. Circulating vascular progenitor cells contribute to vascular repair remodelling and lesion formation. *Trends Cardiovasc Med* 2003; 13: 249–253.

34. Fuster V, et al. Atherothrombosis and high-risk plaque: part 1: evolving concepts. *J Am Coll Cardiol*, September 20, 2005; 46(6): 937–954.

35. Waxman S, Ishibashi F, Muller JE. Detection and treatment of vulnerable plaques and vulnerable patients: novel approaches to prevention of coronary events. *Circulation*, November 28, 2006; 114(22): 2390–2411.

36. Naghavi M, Libby P, Falk E et al. From vulnerable plaque to vulnerable patient: a call for new definitions and risk assessment strategies. Part II, *Circulation* 2003; 108: 1772–1778.

37. Naghavi M, Libby P, Falk E et al. From vulnerable plaque to vulnerable patient: a call for new definitions and risk assessment strategies. Part I, *Circulation* 2003; 108: 1664–1672.

38. Aboyans V, Criqui MH, Deneberg JO et al. Risk factors for progression of peripheral arterial disease in large and small vessels. *Circulation*, June 6, 2006; 113(22): 2623–2629.

39. Ridker PM, Cushman M, Stampfer MJ et al. Inflammation, aspirin and the risk of cardiovascular disease in apparently healthy men. *N Engl J Med*. 1997; 336: 973–979.

40. Turlapaty PDMV, Altura BM. Magnesium deficiency produces spasms of coronary arteries: relationship to aetiology of sudden death ischemic heart disease. *Science* 1980, 208: 198–200.

41. Ueshima K. Magnesium and ischemic heart disease: a review of epidemiological, experimental and clinical evidences. *Magnes Res.* 2005 Dec; 18(4): 275–84.

42. Baird AE. The forgotten lymphocyte: immunity and stroke. *Circulation*, May 2, 2006; 113(17): 2035–2036.

43. Texon M. *Hemodynamic basis for atherosclerosis with critique of the cholesterol-heart disease hypothesis.* Begell House, New York 1995.

44. Burke AP, Kolodgie FD, Farb A et al. Healed plaque ruptures and sudden coronary death, evidence that subclinical rupture has a role in plaque progression. *Circulation.* 2001; 103: 934–940.

45. Falk E, Shah PK, Fuster V. Atherothrombosis and thrombosis-prone plaques. In: Fuster V et al. editors. Hurst's the Heart. 11th edition. New York, NY: McGraw-Hill; 2004. pp. 1123–1139.

46. Ridker PM, Rifai N, Pfeffer M et al. Plasma concentration of interleukin-6 and the risk of future myocardial infarction among apparently healthy men. *Circulation.* 2000; 101: 1767–1772.

47. Libby P. Currant concepts of the pathogenesis of the acute coronary syndromes. *Circulation.* 2001; 104: 365–372.

48. Rosch PJ. Views on Cholesterol. *Health and Stress. The Newsletter of The*

American Institute of Stress, volumes 1995: 1, 1998: 1, 1999: 8, 2001: 2,4,7.

49. Maseri A. From syndromes to specific disease mechanisms. The search for the causes of myocardial infarction. *Ital Heart J.* 2000; 1: 253–257.

50. Matthias R. *Why animals don't get heart attacks – but people do!* MR Publishing, 2000.

51. Alberts et al. *Molecular Biology of the Cell*: 4th edition, NY: Garland Science, 2002.

52. Guyton and Hall (2011). *Textbook of Medical Physiology.* U.S.: Saunders Elsevier.

53. Berg JM, Tymoczko JL and Stryer L. *Biochemistry*, 2006.

54. Mann J, Davies MJ. Mechanisms of progression in native coronary artery disease, role of healed plaque disruption. *Heart* 1999; 82: 265–268.

55. Pinon P, Kaski JC. Inflammation, atherosclerosis and cardiovascular disease risk: PAPP-A, Lp-PLA2 and cystatin C. New insights or redundant information? *Rev Esp Cardio.* 2006 Mar; 59(3): 247–58.

56. Muldoon MF et al. Immune system differences in men with hypo- or hypercholesterolemia. *Clinical Immunology and Immunopathology* 84, 145–149, 1997.

57. Falk E. Multiple culprits in acute coronary syndromes, systemic disease calling for systemic treatment. *Ital Heart J* 2000; 1: 835–838.

58. Glass CK, Witztum JL. Atherosclerosis. The road ahead. *Cell* 2001; 104: 503–516.

59. King JY, Ferrara R, Tabibiazar R et al. Pathway analysis of coronary atherosclerosis. *Physiol Genomics*, September 21, 2005; 23(1): 103–118.

60. Pasceri V, Willerson JT, Yeh ET. Direct proinflammatory effect of C reactive protein on human endothelial cells. *Circulation.* 2000; 102: 2165–2168.

61. Berk BC, Weintraub WS, Alexander RW. Elevation of C-reactive protein in "active" coronary artery disease. *Am J Cardiol.* 1990; 65: 168–172.

62. Mendall MA, Strachan DP, Butland BK et al. C-reactive protein: relation to total mortality, cardiovascular mortality and cardiovascular risk factors in men. *Eur Heart J.* 2000; 21: 1584–1590.

63. Linnemann B, Voigt W, Nobel W, Janka HU. C-reactive protein is a strong independent predictor of death in type 2 diabetes: association with multiple facets of the metabolic syndrome. *Exp Clin Endocrinol Diabetes.* 2006 Mar; 114(3): 127–34.

64. Berliner J, Leitinger N, Watson A et al. Oxidized lipids in atherogenesis: formation, destruction and action. *Thromb Haemost.* 1997; 78: 195–199.

65. Baynes JW, Thorpe SR. Role of oxidative stress in diabetic complications: a new perspective on an old paradigm. *Diabetes.* 1999; 48: 1–9.

66. Cook S. Coronary artery disease, nitric oxide and oxidative stress: the "Yin-Yang" effect – a Chinese concept for a worldwide pandemic. *Swiss Med Wkly*. 2006 Feb 18; 136(7–8): 103–13.
67. Gey KF, Puska P, Jordan P, Moser UK. Inverse correlation between plasma vitamin E and mortality from ischemic heart disease in cross-cultural epidemiology. *American Journal of Clinical Nutrition* 1991, 53: p 326.
68. Pizzorno JE, Murray MT. *Textbook of natural medicine*. 4th edition, 2012.
69. Ginter E. Marginal vitamin C deficiency, lipid metabolism and atherosclerosis. *Lipid Research* 1978. 16: 216–220.
70. Ginter E. Vitamin C deficiency, cholesterol metabolism and atherosclerosis. *Journal of Orthomolecular Medicine*, 1991. 6: 166–173.
71. Sokolov B et al. Ageing, atherosclerosis and ascorbic acid metabolism. *Journal of the American Gerontology Society* 1966. 14: 1239–1260.
72. Mozaffarian D, Katan MB et al. Trans fatty acids and cardiovascular disease. *N Engl J Med*, April 13, 2006; 354(15): 1601–1613.
73. Mozaffarian D. Trans fatty acids – effects on systemic inflammation and endothelial function. *Atheroscler Suppl*. 2006 May; 7(2): 29–32.
74. Lopez-Garcia E, et al. "Consumption of trans fatty acids is related to plasma biomarkers of inflammation and endothelial dysfunction", *Journal of Nutrition*, Mar 2005; 135(3): 562–6.
75. Opie LH. Role of carnitine in fatty acid metabolism of normal and ischemic myocardium. *American Heart Journal*, 1979. 97: 375–388.
76. Giugliano D, Ceriello A, Esposito K. The effects of diet on inflammation: emphasis on the metabolic syndrome. *J Am Coll Cardiol*., August 15, 2006; 48(4): 677–685.

Part Two: What is Atherosclerosis?

What causes atherosclerosis

1. Seeley RR, Stephens TD, Tate P. *Anatomy and physiology*, 2nd edition. Mosby Year Book, 1992.
2. Flammer AJ et al. The assessment of endothelial function: from research into clinical practice. *Circulation*. 2012 Aug 7; 126(6): 753–67.
3. Rubanyi GM. The role of endothelium in cardiovascular homeostasis and diseases. *J Cardiovasc Pharmacol* 1993, 22(suppl 4): S1–S14.
4. Guyton and Hall (2011). *Textbook of Medical Physiology*. U.S.: Saunders Elsevier.
5. Drexler H, Hornig B. Endothelial dysfunction in human disease. *J Mol Cell Cardiol*. 1999 Jan; 31(1): 51–60.
6. Endemann DH, Schiffrin EL. Endothelial dysfunction. *J Am Soc Nephrol*. 2004 Aug; 15(8): 1983–92.

7. Davignon J, Ganz P. Role of endothelial dysfunction in atherosclerosis. *Circulation*. 2004 Jun 15; 109(23 Suppl 1): III27–32. Review

8. Mombouli JV, Vanhoutte PM. Endothelial dysfunction: from physiology to therapy. *J Mol Cell Cardiol*. 1999 Jan; 31(1): 61–74.

9. Ricardo JE, Roberto AN et al. Endothelial dysfunction: a comprehensive appraisal. Review. *Cardiovascular Diabetology*, vol.5, Feb 2006.

10. Epstein SS. *Unreasonable risk*. 2001. Published by Environmental Toxicology, PO Box 11170, Chicago, USA.

11. Eaton DL, Klaassen CD. Principles of Toxicology. In Cassarett & Doull's Toxicology, *The Basic Science of Poisons*. 5th edition. 1996. McGraw-Hill.

12. Davis LE. Drug presentation and prescribing. Chap 3 in *Veterinary Pharmacology and Therapeutics*, 6th edition, 1988 Iowa State Press, Ames.

13. Bronaugh RL & Maibach HI eds. Percutaneous absorption: drugs–cosmetics–mechanisms–methodology, 3rd ed. New York, Marcel Dekker, pp 685–716 (*Drugs and the Pharmaceutical Sciences* Vol. 97).

14. Dressler WE (1999) Hair dye absorption. In: Bronaugh RL & Maibach HI eds. Percutaneous absorption: drugs–cosmetics–mechanisms–methodology, 3rd ed. New York, Marcel Dekker, pp 685–716 (*Drugs and the Pharmaceutical Sciences Vol*. 97).

15. Dang. 1996. EPA SOP. Estimating post application dermally absorbed dose from chemicals in swimming pools.

16. Baynes RE & Hodgson E. Absorption and Distribution of Toxicants. In Chapter 6 of a *Textbook of Modern Toxicology*. 3rd edition. 2004, John Wiley & Sons, Inc.

17. WHO / WMS 2011 – Pharmaceutical Consumption, Annex 3 – Volume Growth in Pharmaceutical Consumption in the Non-hospital Sector, 2000–2008.

18. Andronikashvili I et al. Influence of smoking on endothelial function. *Bul of Georgian N Academy of Sci*, vol. 2, 4, 2008.

19. Esen EM et al. Effect of smoking on endothelial function and wall thickness of brachial artery. *Circulation*, 2004.

20. De Hartog JJ, Hoek G, Peters A, et al. Effects of fine and ultrafine particles on cardiorespiratory symptoms in elderly subjects with coronary heart disease: the ULTRA Study. *Am J Epidemiology* 2003; 157(7): 613–23.

21. Dockery DW, Pope C, Xu X et al. An association between air pollution and mortality in six US cities. *N Eng J Med* 1993; 329(24): 1753–9.

22. Hoek G, Brunekreef B, Fischer P et al. The association between air pollution and heart failure, arrhythmia, embolism, thrombosis and

other cardiovascular causes of death in a time series. *Epidemiology* 2001; 12(3): 355–7.

23. Maynard RL, Howard CV. Air pollution and health. London: Academic Press 1999; 673–705.

24. Xiong X et al. Subchronic toxicity organophosphate insecticide-induced damages on endothelial function of vessels in rabbits by inhibiting antioxidases. *Progress in biochemistry and biophisics*, 2010/37; 11: 1232–1239.

25. Wang P et al. Mechanisms of sodium fluoride-induced endothelial cell barrier dysfunction: role of MLC phosphorylation. *Fluoride 2003*, Vol. 36 No. 1 45–69.

26. Fallon S and Enig M. *Nourishing Traditions: The Cookbook that Challenges Politically Correct Nutrition and the Diet Dictocrats*. 1999. New Trends Publishing.

27. Pizzorno JE, Murray MT. *Textbook of natural medicine*. 4th edition, 2012.

28. Lopez-Garcia E et al. "Consumption of trans fatty acids is related to plasma biomarkers of inflammation and endothelial dysfunction", *Journal of Nutrition*, Mar 2005; 135(3): 562–6.

29. Mozaffarian D. Trans fatty acids – effects on systemic inflammation and endothelial function. *Atheroscler Suppl.* 2006 May; 7(2): 29–32.

30. Danesh J, Collins R, Peto R. Chronic infections and coronary heart disease: is there a link? *Lancet.* 1997; 350: 480–436.

31. Gibson FC, Yumoto H, Takahashi Y et al. Innate immune signalling and porphyromonas gingivalis-accelerated atherosclerosis. *J Dent Res*, February 1, 2006; 85(2): 106–121.

32. Kol A, Bourcier T, Lichtman AH et al. Chlamydial and human heat shock protein 60s activate human vascular endothelium, smooth muscle cells and macrophages. *J Clin Invest.* 1999; 103: 571–577.

33. Libby P, Egan D, Skarlatos S. Roles of infectious agents in atherosclerosis and restenosis: an assessment of the evidence and need for future research. *Circulation.* 1997; 96: 4095–4103.

34. Romano Garratelli C, Nuzzo I, Cozzolino D et al. Relationship between Chlamydia pneumoniae infection, inflammatory markers, and coronary heart disease. *Int Immunopharmacol.* 2006 May; 6(5): 848–53.

35. Virok D, Kis Z, Kari L et al. Chlamydophila pneumoniae and human cytomegalovirus in atherosclerotic carotid plaques – combined presence and possible interactions. *Acta Microbiol Immunol Hung.* 2006 Mar; 53(1): 35–50.

36. Roivanen M, Viik-Kajander M, Paluso T et al. Infections, inflammation and the risk of coronary heart disease. *Circulation.* 2000; 101: 252–257.

37. "NIH Human Microbiome Project". *Genome Res* 19 (12): 2317–2323. 2009.
38. Ley RE, Peterson DA, Gordon JI (2006). "Ecological and Evolutionary Forces Shaping Microbial Diversity in the Human Intestine". *Cell* 124: 837–848.
39. Backhed F, Ley RE, Sonnenburg JL, Peterson DA, Gordon JI (2005). "Host-Bacterial Mutualism in the Human Intestine". *Science* 307: 1915–1920.
40. Salvucci E. (2014). "Microbiome, holobiont and the net of life". *Critical Reviews in Microbiology*: 1.
41. Vinjé SI, Stroes E, Nieuwdorp M, Hazen SL. The gut microbiome as novel cardio-metabolic target: the time has come! *Eur Heart J*. 2014; 35: 883–887.
42. Tilg II. Obesity, metabolic syndrome, and microbiota: multiple interactions. *J Clin Gastroenterol*. 2010; 44 Suppl 1: S16–18.
43. Gori T, Burstein JM et al. Folic acid prevents nitroglycerin-induced nitric oxide sinthase dysfunction and nitrate tolerance. A human in vivo study. *Circulation* 2001, 104: 1119–1123.
44. Münzel T, et al (2008). "Pathophysiology, diagnosis and prognostic implications of endothelial dysfunction". *Annals of Medicine* 40 (18382884): 180–196.
45. Cook S. Coronary artery disease, nitric oxide and oxidative stress: the "Yin-Yang" effect – a Chinese concept for a worldwide pandemic. *Swiss Med Wkly*. 2006 Feb 18; 136(7–8): 103–13.
46. MacReady et al. FLAVURS Study Group (2014). "Flavonoid-rich fruit and vegetables improve microvascular reactivity and inflammatory status in men at risk of cardiovascular disease—FLAVURS: A randomized controlled trial". *American Journal of Clinical Nutrition* 99 (3): 479–89.
47. Selhub, J. (1999). "Homocysteine metabolism". *Annual Review of Nutrition* 19: 217–246.
48. Nygård O at al. (Nov 15, 1995). "Total plasma homocysteine and cardiovascular risk profile. The Hordaland Homocysteine Study." *JAMA: the Journal of the American Medical Association* 274 (19): 1526–33.
49. Berg JM, Tymoczko JL and Stryer L. *Biochemistry*, 2006.
50. Utermann G (1989). "The mysteries of lipoprotein(a)". *Science* 246 (4932): 904–10.
51. Fallon S, Enig M. *Nourishing Traditions. The cookbook that challenges politically correct nutrition and the diet dictocrats*. 1999. New Trends Publishing, Washington DC 20007.
52. BSAEM/BSNM. *Effective Nutritional Medicine: the application of nutrition to major health problems*. 1995. From the British Society for Allergy

Environmental and Nutritional Medicine, PO Box 7 Knighton, LD7 1WT.

53. Vitamin D physiology. *Prog Biophys Mol Biol.* 2006 Sep; 92(1): 4–8. Epub 2006 Feb 28. Review.

54. Heaney RP. The vitamin D requirement in health and disease. *Journal of Steroid Biochemistry & Molecular Biology,* 97 (2005), 13–19.

55. Vitamin D: its role in cancer prevention and treatment. *Prog Biophys Mol Biol.* 2006 Sep; 92(1): 49–59. Epub 2006 Mar 10. Review.

56. Sunlight and vitamin D for bone health and prevention of autoimmune diseases, cancers, and cardiovascular disease. *Am J Clin Nutr.* 2004 Dec; 80(6 Suppl): 1678S–88S. Review.

57. Vitamin D and cancer. *Anticancer Res.* 2006 Jul–Aug; 26(4A): 2515–24. Review.

58. An estimate of premature cancer mortality in the U.S. due to inadequate doses of solar ultraviolet-B radiation. *Cancer.* 2002 Mar 15; 94(6): 1867–75.

59. Beneficial effects of sun exposure on cancer mortality. *Prev Med.* 1993 Jan; 22(1): 132–40. Review.

60. Does sunlight prevent cancer? A systematic review. *Eur J Cancer.* 2006 Sep; 42(14): 2222–32. Epub 2006 Aug 10. Review.

61. Does sunlight have a beneficial influence on certain cancers? *Prog Biophys Mol Biol.* 2006 Sep; 92(1): 132–9. Epub 2006 Feb 28. Review.

62. Ecologic studies of solar UVB radiation and cancer mortality rates. Recent Results. *Cancer Res.* 2003; 164: 371–7. Review.

63. Geographic patterns of prostate cancer mortality. Evidence for a protective effect of ultraviolet radiation. *Cancer.* 1992 Dec 15;70(12):2861–9.

64. Multiple sclerosis and prostate cancer: what do their similar geographies suggest? *Neuroepidemiology.* 1992; 11(4–6): 244–54.

65. UV radiation and cancer prevention: what is the evidence? *Anticancer Res.* 2006 Jul–Aug; 26(4A): 2723–7. Review.

66. Cone JE. Book review on: Toxic Deception: How the Chemical Industry Manipulates Science, Bends the Law, and Endangers your Health, 2nd Edition, by Dan Fagin, Marianne Lavelle and the Centre for Public Integrity. *JAMA* 2000; 283: 121–2.

67. Barnett AH at al. Type 2 diabetes and cardiovascular risk in the UK south Asian community. *Diabetologia* (2006) 49: 2234–2246.

68. Tunstall-Pedoe S et al. Prevention of coronary artery disease: the south Asian paradox. *The Lancet,* 2003.

69. Harris SS et al. Vitamin D and African Americans. *Am Society for Nutrition,* 2006. http://jn.nutrition.org/content/136/4/1126.full

70. Mulukutla SR et al. Black race is associated with digital artery

endothelial dysfunction: results from the Heart SCORE study. *Eur Heart J.* 2010 Nov; 31(22): 2808–15.

71. Davignon J, Ganz P. Role of endothelial dysfunction in atherosclerosis. *Circulation.* 2004 Jun 15; 109(23 Suppl 1): III27–32. Review.

72. "Age related vascular endothelial function following lifelong sedentariness: positive impact of cardiovascular conditioning without further improvement following low frequency high intensity interval training. Physiological Reports" http://physreports.physiology.org/content/3/1/e12234.most-read.

73. Biological Effects of Power Frequency Electric and Magnetic Fields (May 1989, //www.princeton.edu/~ota/disk1/1989/8905/8905.PDF.

74. Atkinson, JLD, Sundt, TM, Dale, AJD et al, Radiation-associated atheromatous disease of the cervical carotid artery: report of seven cases and review of the literature. *Neurosurgery.* 1989; 24: 171–178.

75. Giugliano D, Ceriello A, Esposito K. The effects of diet on inflammation: emphasis on the metabolic syndrome. *J Am Coll Cardiol.*, August 15, 2006; 48(4): 677–685.

76. Hanefeld M, Metzler W, Kohler C, Schaper F. Metabolic syndrome: "common soil" for diabetes and atherosclerosis. Novel approaches to an integrated therapy. *Herz.* 2006 May; 31(3): 246–254.

77. Alberts et al. *Molecular Biology of the Cell*: 4th edition, NY: Garland Science, 2002.

78. Guyton and Hall (2011). *Textbook of Medical Physiology.* U.S.: Saunders Elsevier.

79. Pizzorno JE, Murray MT. *Textbook of natural medicine.* 4th edition, 2012.

80. Garrow JS, James WPT, Ralph A. *Human nutrition and dietetics.* 10th edition. Churchill Livingstone, 2000.

81. WHO global database on obesity, http://apps.who.int/bmi/index.jsp.

82. Modan et al. (March 1985). "Hyperinsulinemia: a link between hypertension, obesity and glucose intolerance". *J. Clin. Invest.* 75 (3): 809–817.

83. Linnemann B, Voigt W, Nobel W, Janka HU. C-reactive protein is a strong independent predictor of death in type 2 diabetes: association with multiple facets of the metabolic syndrome. *Exp Clin Endocrinol Diabetes.* 2006 Mar; 114(3): 127–34.

84. Telkova IL, Tepliakov AT, Karpov RS. The clinical conditions of the manifestation of hyperinsulinemia in patients with coronary heart disease. (Article in Russian). *Klin Med (Mosk).* 2006; 84(4): 18–23.

85. Yudkin JS, Stehouwer CD, Emeis JJ et al. C-reactive protein in healthy subjects: associations with obesity, insulin resistance and endothelial dysfunction: a potential role for cytokines originating from adipose tissue? *Arterioscler Thromb Vasc Biol.* 1999; 19: 972–978.

86. Glass CK, Witztum JL. Atherosclerosis. The road ahead. *Cell* 2001; 104: 503–516.

87. Hansson GK. Inflammation, atherosclerosis and coronary artery disease. *N Engl J Med* 2005; 352: 1685.

88. Vistoli, G et al (Aug 2013). "Advanced glycoxidation and lipoxidation end products (AGEs and ALEs): an overview of their mechanisms of formation." *Free Radic Res.* 47 (12): Suppl 1:3–27.

89. Liuzzo G, Biasucci LM, Gallimore JR et al. The prognostic value of C-reactive protein and serum amyloid A protein in severe unstable angina. *N Engl J Med.* 1997; 331: 417–424.

90. Morrow DA, Rifai N, Antman EM et al. Serum amyloid A predicts early mortality in acute coronary syndromes: a TIMI 11A substudy. *J Am Coll Cardiol.* 2000; 35: 358–362.

91. Glenn J, Stitt A. (2009). "The role of advanced glycation end products in retinal ageing and disease". *Biochimica et Biophysica Acta* 1790 (10): 1109–1116.

92. Gugliucci A, Mehlhaff K, Kinugasa E et al. (2007). "Paraoxonase-1 concentrations in end-stage renal disease patients increase after hemodialysis: correlation with low molecular AGE adduct clearance". *Clin. Chim. Acta* 377 (1–2): 213–20.

93. Miyata et al (September 1993). "beta 2-Microglobulin modified with advanced glycation end products is a major component of hemodialysis-associated amyloidosis.". *The Journal of Clinical Investigation* 92 (3): 1243–52.

94. Sasaki N et al. Advanced glycation end products in Alzheimer's disease and other neurodegenerative diseases. *Am J Pathol* 1998 Oct; 153(4): 1149–55.

95. Feldman HA et al. Impotence and its medical and psychosocial correlates: results of the Massachussetts Male Aging Study. *J Urol.* 1994; 151: 54–61.

96. Vlassara H, Palace MR. Diabetes and advanced glycation endproducts. *J Intern Med.* 2002; 251 (2): 87–101.

97. Gugliucci A. Glycation as the glucose link to diabetic complications. *The Journal of the American Osteopathic Association 2000;* 100 (10): 621–34.

98. Schmidt AM, Yan SD, Wautier JL et al. Activation of receptor for advanced glycation end products: a mechanism for chronic vascular dysfunction in diabetic vasculopathy and atherosclerosis. *Circ Res.* 1999; 84: 489–497.

99. Swaminathan R. "Magnesium Metabolism and its Disorders". US National Library of Medicine National Institutes of Health. Retrieved 31 May 2014.

100. Carolyn Dean. *The Magnesium Miracle.* Ballantine Books, 2007.

101. Nelson DL and Cox MM. *Lehninger Principles of Biochemistry*, 4th edition, 2004.

102. Bilbey DL et al. Muscle cramps and magnesium deficiency: case reports. *Can Fam Physician*. 1996 Jul; 42: 1348–1351.

103. Joffres MR, Reed DM, Yano K. Relationship of magnesium intake and other dietary factors to blood pressure: the Honolulu Heart Study. *Am J Clin Nutr*. 1987; 45: 469–475.

104. Altura BM, Zhang A, Altura BT. Magnesium, hypertensive vascular diseases, atherogenesis, subcellular compartmentation of Ca^{2+} and Mg^{2+} and vascular contractility. *Miner Electrolyte Metab*. 1993; 19: 323–336.

105. Altura BM, Altura BT. Magnesium and cardiovascular biology: an important link between cardiovascular risk factors and atherogenesis. *Cell Mol Biol Res*. 1995; 41: 347–359.

106. Stendig-Lindberg G et al. Sudden death of athletes: is it due to long-term changes in serum magnesium, lipids and blood sugar? *J Basic Clin Physiol Pharmacol*. 1992 Apr–Jun; 3(2): 153–64.

107. Henrotte JG. Type A behaviour and magnesium metabolism. *Magnesium* 5: 201–10, 1986.

108. Kirow GK, Birch NJ, Steadman P, Ramsey RG. Plasma magnesium levels in a population of psychiatric patients: correlation with symptoms *Neuropsychobiology* 30(2–3). 73–8, 1994.

109. Kantak KM. Magnesium deficiency alters aggressive behaviour and catecholamine function. *Behav Neurosci* 102(2): 304–11, 1988.

110. Durlach J. Clinical aspects of chronic magnesium deficiency, in MS Seelig, Ed. *Magnesium in Health and Disease*. New York, Spectrum Publications, 1980.

111. Pizzorno JE, Murray MT. *Textbook of natural medicine*. 4th edition, 2012.

112. Nadler JL et al. Magnesium deficiency produce insulin resistance and increased thromboxane synthesis. *Hypertension*. 1993; 21: 1024–1029.

113. King JY, Ferrara R, Tabibiazar R et al. Pathway analysis of coronary atherosclerosis. *Physiol Genomics*, September 21, 2005; 23(1): 103–118.

Part Three: What To Do?

Step 1: Stop eating processed foods!

1. Common Methods of Processing and Preserving Food. *Streetdirectory. com*. April 7, 2015.

2. Food Processing Lesson Plan. *Johns Hopkins Bloomberg School of Public Health*. April 7, 2015.

3. Levenstein, H: "Paradox of Plenty", p. 106–107. University of California Press, 2003.
4. Most packaged supermarket food is unhealthy – study. http://www.radionz.co.nz/news/national/280056/%27supermarket-food-largely-unhealthy%27.
5. Ultra processed foods prevalent and unhealthy research. http://www.sciencemediacentre.co.nz/2015/07/30/ultra-processed-foods-prevalent-unhealthy-research/.
6. Gracy-Whitman L, Ell S. Artificial colourings and adverse reactions. *BMJ* 1995; 310: 1204.
7. Rogers S. *Tired or toxic? A blueprint for health.* 1990. Prestige Publishers.
8. Rowe KS, Rose KJ. Synthetic food colouring and behaviour: A dose response effect in a double-blind, placebo-controlled, repeated-measures study. *Journal of Paediatrics* 12: 691–698, 1994.
9. Rowe KS. Synthetic food colouring and hyperactivity: a double-blind crossover study. *Aust Paediatr J*, 24: 143–47, 1988.
10. Boris M, Mandel F. Food and additives are common causes of the attention deficit hyperactive disorder in children. *Annals of Allergy* 72: 462–68, 1994.
11. Rea WJ. *Chemical Sensitivity.* Vols. 1,2,3,4. Lewis, Boca Raton, 1994–1998.
12. Guyton and Hall (2011). *Textbook of Medical Physiology.* U.S.: Saunders Elsevier.
13. Garrow JS, James WPT, Ralph A. *Human nutrition and dietetics.* 2000. 10th edition. Churchill Livingstone.
14. Mirkkunen M (1982). Reactive hypoglycaemia tendency among habitually violent offenders. *Neuropsychopharmacol* 8: 35–40.
15. Geary A. *The food and mood handbook.* 2001. Thorsons.
16. Foster-Powell K, Holt SH, Brand-Miller JC. International table of glycemic index and glycemic load values: 2002. *Am J Clin Nutr* 2002; 76: 5–56.
17. Pizzorno JE, Murray MT. *Textbook of natural medicine.* 4th edition, 2012.
18. O'Hara AM, Shanahan F. The gut flora as a forgotten organ. *EMBO reports.* 2006; 7(7): 688–693.
19. MacDougall, Raymond (13 June 2012). "NIH Human Microbiome Project defines normal bacterial makeup of the body". *NIH.* Retrieved 2012–09–20.
20. Eaton KK. Sugars in food intolerance and abnormal gut fermentation. *J Nutr Med* 1992; 3: 295–301.
21. Fayemiwo SA et al. Gut fermentation syndrome. *African J Cl Exp Microbiol*, Vol 15, No 1 (2014).
22. Bivin WS et al. Production of ethanol from infant food formulas by common yeasts. *J Appl Bacteriol*, Vol 58, 4, pp. 355–357, April 1985.

23. Round JL, Mazmanian SK. (2009). "The gut microbiota shapes intestinal immune responses during health and disease". *Nature Reviews: Immunology*, 9(5): 313–323.
24. Yudkin J. *Pure, white and deadly. How sugar is killing us and what we can do to stop it.* 2012.
25. Hurst AF, Knott FA. Intestinal carbohydrate dyspepsia. *Quart J Med* 1930–31; 24: 171–80.
26. Fallon S, Enig M. *Nourishing Traditions. The cookbook that challenges politically correct nutrition and the diet dictocrats.* 1999. New Trends Publishing, Washington DC 20007.
27. Sandstead HH. Fibre, phytates, and mineral nutrition. *Nutr Rev* 1992; 50: 30–1.
28. Freed DL. Lectins in food: their importance in health and disease. *J Nutr Med* 1991; 2: 45–64.
29. Freed DL. Do dietary lectins cause disease? *Br Med J* 1999; 318(71090): 1023–4.
30. Pusztai A, Ewen SW, Grant G et al. Antinutritive effects of wheat-germ agglutinin and other N-acetylglucosamine-specific lectins. *Br J Nutr* 1993; 70: 313–21.
31. Cordain L. Cereal grains: humanity's double-edged sword. *World Rev Nutr Diet* 1999; 84: 19–73.
32. Pizzorno JE, Murray MT. *Textbook of natural medicine.* 4th edition, 2012.
33. Enig MG. *Know Your Fats: The Complete Primer for Understanding the Nutrition of Fats, oils, and Cholesterol.* Bethesda Press, Silver Spring, MD, 2000.
34. Centers for Disease Control and Prevention (1994). "Documentation for Immediately Dangerous To Life or Health Concentrations (IDLHs) – Acrylamide". http://www.cdc.gov/niosh/idlh/79061.html
35. Xu Y et al (Apr 5, 2014). "Risk assessment, formation, and mitigation of dietary acrylamide: Current status and future prospects.". *Food and chemical toxicology: an international journal published for the British Industrial Biological Research Association* 69C: 1–12.
36. Tareke E, Rydberg P et al. (2002). "Analysis of acrylamide, a carcinogen formed in heated foodstuffs". *J. Agric. Food. Chem.* 50 (17): 4998–5006.
37. COMA Report. Dietary sugars and human disease: conclusions and recommendations. *Br Dent J.* 1990; 165: 46.
38. http://www.statista.com/statistics/249681/total-consumption-of-sugar-worldwide/
39. Berg JM, Tymoczko JL and Stryer L. *Biochemistry*, 2006.
40. Tran G., 2015. *Sugarcane press mud.* Feedipedia, a programme by INRA, CIRAD, AFZ and FAO. http://www.feedipedia.org/node/563 *Last updated on May 27, 2015, 18:02.*

41. Dowling RN. (1928). *Sugar Beet and Beet Sugar*. London: Ernest Benn Limited.
42. Altura BM, Zhang A, Altura BT. Magnesium, hypertensive vascular diseases, atherogenesis, subcellular compartmentation of Ca^{2+} and Mg^{2+} and vascular contractility. *Miner Electrolyte Metab*. 1993; 19: 323–336.
43. Altura BM, Altura BT. Magnesium and cardiovascular biology: an important link between cardiovascular risk factors and atherogenesis. Cell Mol Biol Res. 1995; 41: 347–359.
44. Yudkin J. *Pure, white and deadly. How sugar is killing us and what we can do to stop it*. 2012.
45. http://www.sugarstacks.com/beverages.htm
46. Tournas VH et al. Moulds and yeasts in fruit salads and fruit juices. *Food Microbiol*, vol 23; 7, Oct 2006, pp. 684–688.
47. Whysner J, Williams GM (1996). "Saccharin mechanistic data and risk assessment: urine composition, enhanced cell proliferation, and tumour promotion". *Pharmacol Ther* 71 (1–2): 225–52.
48. Lim U, Subar AF, Mouw T et al. Consumption of aspartame-containing beverages and incidence of hematopoietic and brain malignancies. *Cancer Epidemiology, Biomarkers and Prevention* 2006; 15(9): 1654–1659.
49. Roberts HJ (2004). "Aspartame disease: a possible cause for concomitant Graves' disease and pulmonary hypertension". *Texas Heart Institute Journal* 31 (1): 105; author reply 105–6. PMC 387446. PMID 15061638.
50. Humphries P, Pretorius E, Naudé H (2008). "Direct and indirect cellular effects of aspartame on the brain". *Eur J Clin Nutrition* 62 (4): 451–462. doi:10.1038/sj.ejcn.1602866. PMID 17684524.
51. Trocho C, Pardo R, Rafecas I et al. (1998). "Formaldehyde derived from dietary aspartame binds to tissue components in vivo". *Life Sciences* 63 (5): 337–49.
52. Staff writers (March 2010). "The lowdown on high-fructose corn syrup". *Consumer Reports*.
53. Engber D (28 April 2009). "The decline and fall of high-fructose corn syrup". *Slate Magazine*. Slate.com.
54. Enig MG. *Know Your Fats: The Complete Primer for Understanding the Nutrition of Fats, Oils, and Cholesterol*. Bethesda Press, Silver Spring, MD, 2000.
55. BSAEM/BSNM. *Effective Nutritional Medicine: the application of nutrition to major health problems*. 1995. From the British Society for Allergy Environmental and Nutritional Medicine, PO Box 7 Knighton, LD7 1WT.
56. Gupta MK. (2007). *Practical guide for vegetable oil processing*. AOCS Press, Urbana, Illinois

57. Dam H, Sondergaard E. The encephalomalacia producing effect of arachidonic and linoleic acids. *Zeitschrift fur Ernahrungswissenschaft* 2, 217–222, 1962.

58. Pinckney ER. The potential toxicity of excessive polyunsaturates. Do not let the patient harm himself. *American Heart Journal* 85, 723–726, 1973.

59. West CE, Redgrave TG. Reservations on the use of polyunsaturated fats in human nutrition. *Search* 5, 90–96, 1974.

60. McHugh MI et al. Immunosuppression with polyunsaturated fatty acids in renal transplantation. *Transplantation* 24, 263–267, 1977.

61. Alexander JC, Valli VE, Chanin BE. Biological observations from feeding heated corn oil and heated peanut oil to rats. *Journal of Toxicology and Environmental Health* 21, 295–309, 1087.

62. Enig MG. Trans fatty acids in the food supply: a comprehensive report covering 60 years of research. Enig Associates, Inc., Silver Spring, MD, 1993.

63. Emken EA (1984). "Nutrition and biochemistry of trans and positional fatty acid isomers in hydrogenated oils". *Annual Reviews of Nutrition* 4: 339–376.

64. Enig MG, Atal S, Keeney M, Sampugna J (1990). "Isomeric trans fatty acids in the U.S. diet". *Journal of the American College of Nutrition* 9: 471–486.

65. Ascherio A et al (1994). "Trans fatty acids intake and risk of myocardial infarction". *Circulation* 89: 94–101.

66. Ascherio A et al (1999). "Trans fatty acids and coronary heart disease". *New England Journal of Medicine* 340 (25): 1994–1998.

67. Pizzorno JE, Murray MT. *Textbook of natural medicine*. 4th edition, 2012.

68. Daniel KT. *The Whole Soy Story*. 2006. New Trends Publishing.

69. "History of Soy Sauce, Shoyu, and Tamari – Page 1". *soyinfocenter.com*.

70. Endres Joseph G (2001). *Soy Protein Products*. Champaign-Urbana, IL: AOCS Publishing. pp. 43–44.

71. http://www.alkalizeforhealth.net/Lsoy.htm Soy, aluminium and Alzheimer's disease.

72. Shcherbatykh I, Carpenter DO. The Role of Metals in the Etiology of Alzheimer's Disease. *Journal of Alzheimer's Disease*. 2007; 11(2): 191–205.

73. Henkel J (May–June 2000). "Soy: Health Claims for Soy Protein, Question About Other Components". *FDA Consumer* (Food and Drug Administration) 34 (3): 18–20.

74. Messina M, McCaskill-Stevens W, Lampe JW (September 2006). "Addressing the Soy and Breast Cancer Relationship: Review, Commentary, and Workshop Proceedings". *JNCI Journal of the National Cancer Institute* (National Cancer Institute) 98 (18): 1275–1284.

75. Doerge DR, Sheehan DM. Goitrogenic and estrogenic activity of soy isoflavones. *Environ Health Perspect.* 2002 Jun; 110 Suppl 3: 349–53.
76. Song TT, Hendrich S, Murphy PA (1999). "Estrogenic activity of glycitein, a soy isoflavone". *Journal of Agricultural and Food Chemistry* 47(4): 1607–1610.
77. Dendougui Ferial, Schwedt Georg (2004). "In vitro analysis of binding capacities of calcium to phytic acid in different food samples". *European Food Research and Technology* 219 (4).
78. Committee on Food Protection, Food and Nutrition Board, National Research Council (1973). "Phytates". *Toxicants Occurring Naturally in Foods*. National Academy of Sciences. pp. 363–371.
79. Miniello VL et al (2003). "Soy-based formulas and phyto-oestrogens: A safety profile". *Acta Paediatrica* (Wiley-Blackwell) 91 (441): 93–100.
80. Strom BL et al. (2001). "Exposure to soy-based formula in infancy and endocrinological and reproductive outcomes in young adulthood". *JAMA: the Journal of the American Medical Association* (American Medical Association) 286 (7): 807–814.
81. *Seaweeds and their uses in Japan*. Tokai Univ. Press, 165 p.
82. About salt: production. The Salt Manufacturers Association. http://web.archive.org/web/20090409144219/http://www.saltsense. co.uk/aboutsalt-prod02.htm
83. "A brief history of salt". *Time Magazine*. 15 March 1982. Retrieved 11 October 2013.
84. Fallon S, Enig M. *Nourishing Traditions. The cookbook that challenges politically correct nutrition and the diet dictocrats*. 1999. New Trends Publishing, Washington DC 20007.
85. Lopez, Billie Ann. "Hallstatt's White Gold: Salt". *Virtual Vienna Net*. Retrieved 3 March 2013.
86. "Most Americans should consume less sodium". *Salt*. Centers for Disease Control and Prevention. Retrieved 17 October 2013.
87. "References on food salt & health issues". Salt Institute. 2009. Retrieved 5 December 2010.
88. Strazzullo et al (2009). "Salt intake, stroke, and cardiovascular disease: meta-analysis of prospective studies". *British Medical Journal* 339 (b4567).
89. He FJ, Li J, Macgregor GA (3 April 2013). "Effect of longer term modest salt reduction on blood pressure: Cochrane systematic review and meta-analysis of randomised trials.". *BMJ (Clinical research ed.)* 346: f1325.
90. Graudal NA, Hubeck-Graudal T, Jurgens G (9 November 2011). "Effects of low sodium diet versus high sodium diet on blood pressure, renin, aldosterone, catecholamines, cholesterol, and triglyceride.". *The Cochrane database of systematic reviews* (11): CD004022.

91. Stolarz-Skrzypek K, Staessen JA (March 2015). "Reducing salt intake for prevention of cardiovascular disease—times are changing." *Advances in chronic kidney disease* 22 (2): 108–15.
92. Guyton and Hall (2011). *Textbook of Medical Physiology.* U.S.: Saunders Elsevier.
93. Pizzorno JE, Murray MT. *Textbook of natural medicine.* 4ᵗʰ edition, 2012.

What should we eat to prevent atherosclerosis and its deadly complications?

1. http://www.curezone.org/foods/microwave_oven_risk.asp Microwave oven. The hidden hazards.
2. http://www.naturalnews.com/030651_microwave_cooking_cancer.html Why and how microwave cooking causes cancer.
3. Garrow JS, James WPT, Ralph A. *Human nutrition and dietetics.* 2000. 10ᵗʰ edition. Churchill Livingstone.
4. Kleinbongard P et al (2006). "Plasma nitrite concentrations reflect the degree of endothelial dysfunction in humans". *Free Radical Biology and Medicine* 40 (2): 295–302.
5. "Additives Used in Meat". *Meat Science.* Illinois State University. Retrieved 16 December 2010.
6. Nutrient composition of chicken meat. 2009 Rural Industries Research and Development Corporation. ISBN 1 74151 799 0, ISSN 1440-6845.
7. Ensimger AH et al. *The Concise Encyclopedia of Food and Nutrition.* CRC Press, 1995.
8. Pizzorno JE, Murray MT. *Textbook of natural medicine.* 4ᵗʰ edition, 2012.
9. Stipanuk MH. (2006). *Biochemical, Physiological and Molecular Aspects of Human Nutrition* (2nd ed.). Philadelphia: Saunders.
10. Masterjohn C. On the trail of the elusive x factor: a sixty-two-year-old mystery finally solved. *Wise Traditions.* 2007; 8(1).
11. Vormann J, Daniel H. The role of nutrition in human acid-base homeostasis. *Eur J Nutr* 2001; 40: 187–8.
12. Fallon S, Enig M. *Nourishing Traditions. The cookbook that challenges politically correct nutrition and the diet dictocrats.* 1999. New Trends Publishing, Washington DC 20007.
13. Cordain J, Eaton SB, Miller JB, Mann N, Hill K. The paradoxical nature of hunter-gatherer diets: meat-based, yet non-atherogenic. *Eur J Clin Nutr* 2002; 56(Suppl.1): S42–52.
14. Daniel KT, "Why Broth is Beautiful: Essential Roles for Proline, Glycine and Gelatin," Weston A. Price Foundation. http://www.westonaprice. org/food-features/why-broth-is-beautiful (accessed 18 June 2013).

15. Gottschall E. *Breaking the vicious cycle. Intestinal health through diet.* 1996. The Kirkton Press.
16. Fish consumption advice from USA government. http://www.epa.gov/mercury/advisories.htm
17. Bjornberg KA, Vahter M, Grawé KP, Berglund M (2005). "Methyl Mercury Exposure in Swedish Women with High Fish Consumption". *Science of the Total Environment* 341 (1–3): 45–52.
18. Rowland IR, Grasso P, Davies MJ. The methylation of mercuric chloride by human intestinal bacteria. *Experientia.* 1975 Sep 15; 31(9): 1064–5.
19. Prakash, Satya et al (2011). "Gut microbiota: next frontier in understanding human health and development of biotherapeutics". *Biologics: Targets and Therapy* 5: 71–86.
20. FDA/EPA (2004). "What You Need to Know About Mercury in Fish and Shellfish". Retrieved October 25, 2006.
21. Mercury Levels in Commercial Fish and Shellfish (1990–2010). United States Food and Drug Administration. Retrieved July 1, 2011.
22. Serhan CN, Chiang N, Van Dyke TE. Resolving inflammation: dual anti-inflammatory and pro-resolution lipid mediators. *Nat Rev Immunol.* 2008 May; 8(5): 349–61.
23. Pedersen MH, Molgaard C, Hellgren LI, Lauritzen L. Effects of fish oil supplementation on markers of the metabolic syndrome. *J Pediatr.* 2010 Sep; 157(3): 395–400.
24. Garrow JS, James WPT, Ralph A. *Human nutrition and dietetics.* 2000. 10th edition. Churchill Livingstone.
25. Pizzorno JE, Murray MT. Textbook of natural medicine. 4th edition, 2012.
26. Roy Porter. *The Greatest Benefit to Mankind: A Medical History of Humanity.* 1999.
27. Gray N. "No link between eggs and heart disease or stroke, says BMJ meta-analysis." January 25, 2013. foodnavigator.com/Science/No-link-between-eggs-and-heart-disease-or-stroke-says-BMJ-meta-analysis
28. Ensimger AH et al. *The Concise Encyclopedia of Food and Nutrition.* CRC Press, 1995.
29. Sies H. Antioxidants in disease mechanisms and therapy. *Adv Pharmacol Vol* 38, San Diego: Academic Press, 1997.
30. Irons R. Pasteurization Does Harm Real Milk. realmilk.com/health/pasteurization-does-harm-real-milk/
31. Palupi E, Jayanegara A, Ploeger A, Kahl J (November 2012). "Comparison of nutritional quality between conventional and organic dairy products: a meta-analysis". *J. Sci. Food Agric.* 92 (14): 2774–81.

32. Enig MG. *Know Your Fats: The Complete Primer for Understanding the Nutrition of Fats, Oils, and Cholesterol.* Bethesda Press, Silver Spring, MD, 2000.

33. Oster K, Oster J, Ross D. "Immune Response to Bovine Xanthine Oxidase in Atherosclerotic Patients." *American Laboratory*, August, 1974, 41–47.

34. Perkin MR. Unpasteurized milk: health or hazard? *Clinical and Experimental Allergy* 2007 May; 35(5) 627–630.

35. Waser M, Michels KB, Bieli C et al. Inverse association of farm milk consumption with asthma and allergy in rural and suburban populations across Europe. *Clinical Exp Allergy* 2007; 37:661–70.

36. realmilk.com/real-milk-finder/

37. nhs.uk/conditions/Lactose-intolerance/Pages/Introduction.aspx

38. O'Hara AM, Shanahan F (2006). "The gut flora as a forgotten organ. EMBO reports", 7 (7): 688–693.

39. Gottschall E. *Breaking the vicious cycle. Intestinal health through diet.* 1996. The Kirkton Press.

40. Kris-Etherton PM et al (1999). "Nuts and their bioactive constituents: effects on serum lipids and other factors that affect disease risk". *Am J Clin Nutr* 70 (3 Suppl): 504S–511S.

41. Sabaté J et al (1993). "Effects of walnuts on serum lipid levels and blood pressure in normal men". *Engl J Med* 328 (9): 603–607.

42. Kelly JH, Sabaté J (2006). "Nuts and coronary heart disease: an epidemiological perspective". *Br J Nutr* 96: S61–S67.

43. Dreher ML, Maher CV, Kearney P. The traditional and emerging role of nuts in healthful diets. *Nutr Rev* 1996; 54: 241–5.

44. Campbell-McBride N. *Gut and psychology syndrome. Natural treatment for autism, dyspraxia, dyslexia, ADD/ADHD, depression and schizophrenia.* 2010. Medinform Publishing.

45. Fallon S, Enig M. *Nourishing Traditions. The cookbook that challenges politically correct nutrition and the diet dictocrats.* 1999. New Trends Publishing, Washington DC, 20007.

46. Els JM Van Damme et al. (1998). *Handbook of Plant Lectins: Properties and Biomedical Applications.* John Wiley & Sons.

47. Enig MG. *Know Your Fats: The Complete Primer for Understanding the Nutrition of Fats, Oils, and Cholesterol.* Bethesda Press, Silver Spring, MD, 2000.

48. BSAEM/BSNM. Effective Nutritional Medicine: the application of nutrition to major health problems. 1995. From the British Society for Allergy Environmental and Nutritional Medicine, PO Box 7 Knighton, LD7 1WT.

49. Pizzorno JE, Murray MT. *Textbook of natural medicine.* 4th edition, 2012.

50. Horrobin D. *The madness of Adam and Eve*. Bantam Press. ISBN 0 593 04649 8, 2001.
51. Nelson GJ et al (1997). "The effect of dietary arachidonic acid on plasma lipoprotein distributions, apoproteins, blood lipid levels, and tissue fatty acid composition in humans". *Lipids* 32 (4): 427–33.
52. Kelley DS et al (1998). "Arachidonic acid supplementation enhances synthesis of eicosanoids without suppressing immune functions in young healthy men". *Lipids* 33 (2): 125–30.
53. Gupta MK. (2007). *Practical guide for vegetable oil processing*. AOCS Press, Urbana, Illinois
54. Dam H, Sondergaard E. The encephalomalacia producing effect of arachidonic and linoleic acids. *Zeitschrift fur Ernahrungswissenschaft* 2, 217–222, 1962.
55. Pinckney ER. The potential toxicity of excessive polyunsaturates. Do not let the patient harm himself. *American Heart Journal* 85, 723–726, 1973.
56. West CE, Redgrave TG. Reservations on the use of polyunsaturated fats in human nutrition. *Search* 5, 90–96, 1974.
57. McHugh MI et al. Immunosuppression with polyunsaturated fatty acids in renal transplantation. *Transplantation* 24, 263–267, 1977.
58. Alexander JC, Valli VE, Chanin BE. Biological observations from feeding heated corn oil and heated peanut oil to rats. *Journal of Toxicology and Environmental Health* 21, 295–309, 1087.
59. Ravnskov U. *The Cholesterol Myths. Exposing the fallacy that saturated fat and cholesterol cause heart disease*. 2000. NewTrends Publishing.
60. Garrow JS, James WPT, Ralph A. *Human nutrition and dietetics*. 2000. 10th edition. Churchill Livingstone.
61. Els JM Van Damme et al. (March 30, 1998). Handbook of Plant Lectins: Properties and Biomedical Applications. John Wiley & Sons.
62. Shechter Y. Bound lectins that mimic insulin produce persistent insulin-like activities. *Endocrinology* 1983: 113: 1921–6.
63. Sandstead HH. Fibre, phytates, and mineral nutrition. *Nutr Rev* 1992; 50: 30–1.
64. Elli L et al. (2015). "Diagnosis of gluten related disorders: celiac disease, wheat allergy and non-celiac gluten sensitivity". *World J Gastroenterol*, 21 (23): 7110–9.
65. Smith MW, Phillips AD. Abnormal expression of dipeptidyl peptidase IV activity in enterocyte brush-border membranes of children suffering from celiac disease. *Exp Physiol* 1990 Jul; 75(4); 613–6.
66. Map of Life – "Gut fermentation in herbivorous animals". University of Cambridge. October 27, 2015. http://www.mapoflife.org/topics/topic_206_Gut-fermentation-in-herbivorous-animals/

67. Steinkraus KH, Ed. (1995). *Handbook of Indigenous Fermented Foods.* New York, Marcel Dekker, Inc.
68. Ulijaszek S, Strickland SS. *Nutritional Anthropology: Prospects and Perspectives.* London: Smith-Gordon, 1993.
69. Fallon S, Enig M. Nourishing Traditions. The cookbook that challenges politically correct nutrition and the diet dictocrats. 1999. New Trends Publishing, Washington DC, 20007.
70. Campbell-McBride N. *Gut and psychology syndrome. Natural treatment for autism, dyspraxia, dyslexia, ADD/ADHD, depression and schizophrenia.* 2010. Medinform Publishing.
71. Cooper RA, Molan PC and Harding KG. The sensitivity to honey of Gram-positive cocci of clinical significance isolated from wounds. *Journal of Applied Microbiology*, 93, 857–863 (2002).
72. Honey: health benefits and uses in medicine. http://www.medical-newstoday.com/articles/264667.php
73. Honey kills antibiotic-resistant bugs. Published online 19 November 2002 | *Nature.* doi:10.1038/news021118-1.
74. Herman AC et al. Effect of honey on nocturnal cough and sleep quality: a double-blind, randomized, placebo controlled study. *Pediatrics* Volume 130, Number 3, September 2012.
75. Honey holds some promise for treating burns. Published: 9 October 2008, http://www.hbns.org
76. Haffejee IE, Moosa A. Honey in the treatment of infantile gastroenteritis. *Br Med J (Clin Res Ed)* 1985; 290: 1866.
77. Oesophagus: heartburn and honey. Clinical review. *BMJ* 2001; 323: 736.
78. Oduwole O, Meremikwu MM, Oyo-Ita A, Udoh EE (2014). "Honey for acute cough in children". *Cochrane Database Syst Rev* (Systematic review) 3 (12): CD007094.
79. Majtan, J (2014). "Honey: an immunomodulator in wound healing". *Wound Repair Regen.* 22 (2 Mar–Apr): 187–192.
80. Al-Sahib W and Marshall RJ. "The fruit of the date palm: its possible use as the best food for the future?" *J Food Science Nutr* 2003; 54: 247–59.
81. Carughi A. "Health Benefits of Sun-Dried Raisins". http://www.raisins.net/Raisins_and_Health_200810.pdf
82. Grivetti LE and Applegate EA. "From Olympia to Atlanta: agricultural-historic perspective on diet and athletic training". *J Clinical Nutr* 1997; 127: S860–868.
83. Hooshmand S and Arjmandi BH. "Viewpoint: dried plum, an emerging functional food that may effectively improve bone health". *Ageing Res Reviews* 2009; 8: 122-7.

84. Slavin JL (July–August 2006). *"Figs: past, present and future"*. *Nutrition Today* 41 (4): 180–184.
85. Steinkraus KH Ed. (1995). *Handbook of Indigenous Fermented Foods.* New York, Marcel Dekker, Inc.
86. Murray MT. *The complete book of juicing.* 2014. Random House.
87. Gerson C with Bishop B. *Healing the Gerson way. Defeating cancer and other chronic diseases.* 2007. Totality Books.
88. BSAEM/BSNM. *Effective Nutritional Medicine: the application of nutrition to major health problems.* 1995. From the British Society for Allergy Environmental and Nutritional Medicine, PO Box 7 Knighton, LD7 1WT.
89. Pizzorno JE, Murray MT. *Textbook of natural medicine.* 4th edition, 2012.
90. "The Real Reasons Juice Cleanses Can Get Your Health Back on Track". awaken.com. Retrieved 7 May 2015.
91. Benachour N, Aris A. 2009. Toxic effects of low doses of bisphenol-A on human placental cells. *Toxicology and Applied Pharmacology* 241: 322–8.
92. Brede C, Fjeldal P, Skjevrak I et al. 2003. Increased migration levels of bisphenol A from polycarbonate baby bottles after dishwashing, boiling and brushing. *Food Additives & Contaminants: Part A* 20(7): 684–9.
93. Braun JM, Kalkbrenner AE, Calafat AM et al. 2011. Impact of early-life bisphenol A exposure on behaviour and executive function in children. *Pediatrics* 128(5): 873–882 http://pediatrics.aappublications.org [Accessed September 2014].
94. CPSC. 2011. *FAQs: Bans on phthalates in toys.* Consumer Product Safety Commission (US). www.cpsc.gov [Accessed September 2014].
95. Diamanti-Kandarakis E, Bourguignon JP, Guidice LC et al. 2009. Endocrine-disrupting chemicals: an Endocrine Society scientific statement. *Endocrine* Reviews 30(4): 293–342. www.endo-society.org [Accessed September 2014].
96. Juliano LM, Griffiths RR (2004). "A critical review of caffeine withdrawal: empirical validation of symptoms and signs, incidence, severity, and associated features". *Psychopharmacology* 176 (1): 1–29.
97. Mihaljev Z et al. Levels of some microelements and essential heavy metals in herbal teas in Serbia. *Acta Pol Pharm.* 2014 May–Jun; 71(3): 385–91.
98. Heavy metal contents in tea and herb leaves. *Pakistan J Biol Sciences.* 2003, Vol 6; 3, 2088–212.
99. Vartanian LR, Schwartz MB, Brownell KD. Effects of soft drink consumption on nutrition and health: a systematic review and meta-analysis. *Am J Public Health.* 2007;97:667–75.
100. Malik VS et al. Sugar-sweetened beverages and risk of metabolic

syndrome and type 2 diabetes: a meta-analysis. *Diabetes Care.* 2010; 33: 2477–83.

101. De Koning L et al. Sweetened beverage consumption, incident coronary heart disease, and biomarkers of risk in men. *Circulation.* 2012; 125: 1735–41, S1.
102. Couzin J (2007). "Souring on Fake Sugar". *Science* 317 (5834): 29c.
103. Puddey IB et al. Alcohol and endothelial function: a brief review. *Clin Exp Pharmacol Physiol.* 2001 Dec;28(12):1020–4.
104. Bamforth CW (17–20 September 2006). "Beer as liquid bread: Overlapping science.". World Grains Summit 2006: Foods and Beverages. San Francisco, California, USA.

Step 2: Stop polluting your body!

1. Toxic chemicals in building materials. An overview for health care organizations. http://healthybuilding.net/uploads/files/toxic-chemicals-in-building-materials.pdf [Accessed October 2015]
2. Agocs MA, Etzel RA, Parrish RG et al. Mercury exposure from interior latex paint. *N Engl Med J* 1990; 323: 1096–101.
3. Ashford N, Miller C. *Chemical exposures: low levels and high stakes*, 2nd edn. New York. Van Nostrand Reinhold, 1998.
4. Cone JE. Book review on: *Toxic deception: how the chemical industry manipulates science, bends the law, and endangers your health*, 2nd edition, by Dan Fagin, Marianne Lavelle and the Centre for Public Integrity. *JAMA* 2000; 283: 121–2.
5. Anthony H, Birtwistle S, Eaton K, Maberly J. *Environmental Medicine in Clinical Practice.* BSAENM Publications 1997.
6. http://wellnessmama.com/6244/natural-cleaning-tips/ http://www.keeperofthehome.org/2013/06/homemade-all-natural-cleaning-recipes.html
7. Baghurst PA, McMichael AJ, Wigg NR et al. Environmental exposure to lead and children's intelligence at the age of seven years. The Port Pirie Cohort Study. *N Engl J Med* 1992; 327: 1279–84.
8. Bell I, Miller C, Schwartz G et al. Neuropsychiatric and somatic characteristics of young adults with and without self-reported chemical odour intolerance and chemical sensitivity. *Arch Environ Health* 1996; 51: 9–21.
9. Eaton KK, Anthony HM, Birtwistle S, Downing D, Freed DLJ et al. Multiple chemical sensitivity: recognition and management. A document on the health effects of everyday chemical exposures and their implications. *J Nutr Envir Med* 2000; 10: 39–84.
10. Epstein SS. *Unreasonable risk.* 2001. Published by Environmental Toxicology, PO Box 11170, Chicago, USA.

11. Alfrey AC. Aluminium intoxication. *N Engl J Med* 1984; 310: 1113–1114.
12. Rogers S. *Tired or toxic.* 1990. Prestige Publishers.
13. Aksglaede L, Juul A, Leffers H, Skakkebaek NE, Andersson AM (2006). "The sensitivity of the child to sex steroids: possible impact of exogenous estrogens". *Hum. Reprod.* Update 12 (4): 341–9.
14. Mueller SO (February 2004). "Xenoestrogens: mechanisms of action and detection methods". *Anal Bioanal Chem* 378 (3): 582–7.
15. Clarkson T. Methylmercury toxicity to the mature and developing nervous system: possible mechanisms. In: Sakar B. ed. *Biological Aspects of metals and metal-related diseases.* New York: 1983: 183–197.
16. Farrow A, Taylor H, Golding J. Symptoms of mothers and infants, level of measured volatile organic compounds and use of aerosols and air fresheners. Proceedings of the Indoor Air Conference, Edinburgh, 1999; 2: 286–91.
17. Department of the Environment, Transport and the Regions (DETR). Sustainable Production and Use of Chemicals: Consultation Paper on Chemicals in the Environment. London: DETR, 1998.
18. Gertig DM, Hunter DJ, Cramer DW et al. Prospective study of talc use and ovarian cancer. *J Natl Cancer Inst.* 2000; 92: 249–252.
19. "Final report on the safety assessment of sodium laureth sulfate and ammonium laureth sulfate". *Journal of the American College of Toxicology* 2 (5): 1–34. 1983.
20. Agner T (1991). "Susceptibility of atopic dermatitis patients to irritant dermatitis caused by sodium lauryl sulphate". *Acta Dermato-venereologica* 71 (4): 296–300.
21. http://fluoridealert.org/issues/health/
22. Carbon black, titanium dioxide and talc. WHO International Agency for Research of Cancer. *Monographs on evaluation of carcinogenic risk for humans.* 2010. Vol. 93.
23. Knaak JB et al. Toxicology of mono-, di-, and triethanolamine. *Rev Environ Contam Toxicol.* 1997; 149:1–86.
24. Epstein SS. *Unreasonable risk.* 2001. Published by Environmental Toxicology, PO Box 11170, Chicago, USA.
25. Reuber MD. Carcinogenicity of saccharin. *Environ Health Perspect.* 1978 Aug; 25: 173–200.
26. http://www.health-report.co.uk/ethylene_glycol_propylene_glycol. htm
27. Mench U, Lowenthal RM, Coleman D. Lead poisoning masquerading as chronic fatigue syndrome. *Lancet* 1996; 347: 1193.
28. Apostolidis S et al (2002). "Evaluation of carcinogenic potential of two nitro-musk derivatives, musk xylene and musk tibetene in a host-mediated in vivo/in vitro assay system". *Anticancer Res.* 22 (5): 2657–62.

29. Cone JE. Book review on: *Toxic deception: how the chemical industry manipulates science, bends the law, and endangers your health*, 2nd edition, by Dan Fagin, Marianne Lavelle and the Centre for Public Integrity. JAMA 2000;283:121–2.
30. http://www.health.ny.gov/environmental/emergency/chemical_terrorism/chlorine_tech.htm
31. http://www.permaculture.co.uk/articles/ecological-and-health-benefits-natural-swimming-pools
32. http://articles.mercola.com/sites/articles/archive/2015/01/06/cell-phone-use-brain-cancer-risk.aspx
33. Schnare DW, Ben M, Shields MG. Body burden of PCBs, PBBs and chlorinated pesticides in human subjects. *Ambio* 1984; 13: 378–80.
34. White R, Proctor S. Solvents and neurotoxicity. *Lancet* 1997; 349 (9060) 1239–43.
35. Barnard C. *50 ways to a healthy heart*. 2001. Ozonex Ltd, London, UK.
36. US Public Health Service, Office of the Surgeon General. Physical Activity and Health: A Report of the Surgeon General. Atlanta, GA: US Department of Health and Human Services, Centers for Disease Control and Prevention, National Center for Chronic Disease Prevention and Health Promotion; 1996.
37. Belyaev L. Non-thermal biological effects of microwaves. *Microwave Review*. November 2005, 13–29.

Part Four: All Diseases Begin in the Gut!

1. O'Hara AM and Shanahan F (2006). "The gut flora as a forgotten organ. EMBO reports", 7 (7): 688 693.
2. MacDougall R (13 June 2012). "NIH Human Microbiome Project defines normal bacterial makeup of the body". *NIH*. Retrieved 2012-09-20.
3. Anthony H, Birtwistle S, Eaton K, Maberly J. *Environmental Medicine in Clinical Practice*. BSAENM Publications 1997.
4. Finegold SM, Sutter VL, Mathisen GE (1983). Normal indigenous intestinal flora in *"Human intestinal flora in health and disease"* (Hentges DJ, ed), pp3–31. Academic press, London, UK.
5. Gibson GR, Roberfroid MB (1999). Colonic Microbiota, Nutrition and Health. Kluwer Academic Publishers, Dodrecht.
6. Krasnogolovez VN. *Colonic dysbacteriosis*. M: Medicina, 1989.
7. Petrovskaja VG, Marko OP. *Human microflora in norm and pathology*. M: Medicina, 1976.
8. Roberfroid MB, Bornet F, Bouley C, Cummings JH (1995). Colonic microflora: nutrition and health. Summary and conclusions of an International Life Sciences Institute (ILSI) [Europe] workshop held in

Barcelona, Spain. [Review][33 refs]. *Nutrition Reviews.* 53(5): 127–30, 1995 May.

9. Survey shows link between antibiotics and developmental delays in children. Townsend Letter for Doctors and Patients. October 1995.
10. Samonis G et al. (1994). Prospective evaluation of the impact of broad-spectrum antibiotics on the yeast flora of the human gut. *European Journal of Clinical Microbiology and Infectious Diseases,* 13: 665–7.
11. Falliers C. Oral contraceptives and allergy. *Lancet* 1974; part 2: 515.
12. Grant E. The contraceptive pill: its relation to allergy and illness. *Nutrition and Health* 1983; 2: 33–40.
13. McLaren Howard J. Intestinal dysbiosis. Complementary Therapies. *Med* 1993; 1: 153.
14. Howard J. The "autobrewery" syndrome. *J Nutr Med* 1991; 2: 97–8.
15. Vorobiev AA, Pak SG et al (1998). *Dysbacteriosis in children. A textbook for doctors and medical students.*(Russian). M: "KMK Lt.", 1998. ISBN 5-87317-049-5.
16. Turnbaugh PJ et al. "An obesity-associated gut microbiome with increased capacity for energy harvest." *Nature* 444.7122 (2006): 1027–131.
17. Turnbaugh PJ et al. "A core gut microbiome in obese and lean twins." *Nature* 457.7228 (2009): 480–484.
18. Tang WH et al. Intestinal Microbial Metabolism of Phosphatidlycholine and Cardiovascular Risk. *New England Journal of Medicine* 2013; 368(17): 1575–84.
19. Vinjé SI, Stroes E, Nieuwdorp M, Hazen SL. The gut microbiome as novel cardio-metabolic target: the time has come! *Eur Heart J.* 2014; 35: 883–887.
20. Tilg H. Obesity, metabolic syndrome, and microbiota: multiple interactions. *J Clin Gastroenterol.* 2010; 44 Suppl 1: S16–18.
21. Round J L and Mazmanian SK (2009). "The gut microbiota shapes intestinal immune responses during health and disease". *Nature Reviews: Immunology,* 9 (5): 313–323.
22. Summers AO et al. Mercury released from dental silver fillings provokes an increase in mercury and antibiotic-resistant bacteria in oral and intestinal floras of primates. *Antimicrobial Agents and Chemotherapy,* 1993: 37(4): 825–34.
23. Sullivan NM, Mills DC, Riemann HP, Arnon SS. Inhibitions of growth of Clostridium botulinum by intestinal microflora isolated from healthy infants. *Microbial Ecology in Health and Disease,* 1988; 1:179–92.
24. Wilson K, Moore L, Patel M, Permoad P. Suppression of potential pathogens by a defined colonic microflora. *Microbial Ecology in Health and Disease.* 1988; 1: 237–43.

25. Cummings JH, Macfarlane GT (1997). Role of intestinal bacteria in nutrient metabolism.(Review)(104 refs). *Journal of Parenteral & Enteral Nutrition*.1997, 21(6): 357–65.

26. Cummings JH, Macfarlane GT (1997). Colonic Microflora: Nutrition and Health. *Nutrition.* 1997; vol.13, No. 5, 476–478.

27. Cummings JH (1984). Colonic absorption: the importance of short chain fatty acids in man. (Review)(95refs). *Scandinavian Journal of Gastroenterology* – Supplement. 93: 89–99, 1984.

28. Bjarnason I et al. Intestinal permeability, an overview. (Review). *Gastroenterology*, 1995; 108: 1566–81.

29. Gardner MLG (1994). Absorption of intact proteins and peptides. In: *Physiology of the Gastrointestinal Tract*, 3rd edn. Chapter 53, pp 1795–1820. NY:Raven Press.

30. Troncone R et al. (1987). Passage of gliadin into human breast milk. *Acta Paed Scand*, 76: 453–456.

31. Kilshaw PJ and Cant AJ (1984). The passage of maternal dietary protein into human breast milk. *Int Arch Allergy and Appl Immunol* 75: 8–15.

32. Finegold SM, Sutter VL, Mathisen GE (1983). Normal indigenous intestinal flora in "Human intestinal flora in health and disease" (Hentges DJ, ed), pp. 3–31. Academic Press, London, UK.

33. Gibson GR, Roberfroid MB (1999). Colonic Microbiota, Nutrition and Health. Kluwer Academic Publishers, Dodrecht.

34. Nygård O et al (Nov 15, 1995). "Total plasma homocysteine and cardiovascular risk profile. The Hordaland Homocysteine Study.". *JAMA: the Journal of the American Medical Association* 274 (19): 1526–33.

35. Geleijnse et al. (Nov 1 2004) "Dietary intake of menaquinone is associated with a reduced risk of coronary heart disease: the Rotterdam Study", *J. Nutr.* Vol.134 No.11 pp. 3100–3105, The American Society for Nutritional Sciences.

36. Vorobiev AA, Nesvizski UV (1997). Human microflora and immunity. Review (Russian), *Sovremennie Problemi Allergologii, Klinicheskoi Immunologii i Immunofarmacologii.* M. 1997. c.137–141.

37. Yasui H, Shida K, Matsuzaki T, Yokokuta T (1999). Immuno-modulatory function of lactic acid bacteria. (Review)(28 refs), Antonie van Leenwenhoek. 76(1–4): 38309, 1999 Jul–Nov.

38. Mackie RM. Intestinal permeability and atopic disease. *Lancet* 1981; I: 155.

39. Penders J, Stobberingh EE, van den Brandt PA and Thijs C (2007). "The role of the intestinal microbiota in the development of atopic disorders". *Allergy*, 62 (11): 1223–1236.

40. Steinkraus KH. Ed. (1995). Handbook of Indigenous Fermented Foods. New York, Marcel Dekker, Inc.

41. Ulijaszek S, Strickland SS. Nutritional Anthropology: Prospects and Perspectives. London: Smith-Gordon, 1993.
42. Fallon S, Enig M. *Nourishing Traditions. The cookbook that challenges politically correct nutrition and the diet dictocrats.* 1999. New Trends Publishing, Washington DC, 20007.
43. Cunningham-Rundles S et al (2000). Probiotics and immune response. *American Journal of Gastroenterology,* 95(1 Suppl): S22-5, 2000 Jan.
44. Dunne C et al. 1999. Probiotics: from myth to reality. Demonstration of functionality in animal models of disease and in human clinical trials. (Review)(79 refs). Antonie van Leenwenhoek. 76(104): 279–92, 1999 Jul–Nov.
45. Fuller R. Probiotics in man and animals. *J Appl Bacteriol,* 1989; 66: 365–78.
46. Lewis SJ, Freedman AR (1998). Review article: the use of biotherapeutic agents in the prevention and treatment of gastrointestinal disease. (Review)(144 refs). *Alimentary Pharmacology and Therapeutics.* 12(9): 807–22, 1998 Sep.
47. Rolfe RD. The role of probiotic cultures in the control of gastrointestinal health. *J Nutr,* 2000 Feb; 130(2S) Suppl: 396S–402S Journal Code: JEV.
48. Campbell-McBride N. *Gut and psychology syndrome. Natural treatment for autism, dyspraxia, dyslexia, ADD/ADHD, depression and schizophrenia.* 2010. Medinform Publishing.

There is none so blind as the double blind!

1. Journal-neo.org/2015/06/18/shocking-report-from-medical-insiders/
2. DeGrandpre R. The Cult of Pharmacology. Review. *J Scient Expl,* 21(2), 429–431 (2006).
3. Diamond DM, Ravnskov U. How statistical deception created the appearance that statins are safe and effective in primary and secondary prevention of cardiovascular disease. *Expert Review of Clinical Pharmacology,* 2015 Mar 8(2): 201–210.
4. Kauffman J. *Malignant Medical Myths: Why Medical Treatment Causes 200,000 Deaths in the USA each Year, and How to Protect Yourself.* 2006, Infinity Publishing.
5. Smith R: The Trouble with Medical Journals. *Royal Society of Medicine Press, London,* England 2006.
6. Goldacre B. *Bad Pharma: How Drug Companies Mislead Doctors and Harm Patients.* 2013, Faber & Faber.

Recommended reading

1. Campbell-McBride N. *Gut And Psychology Syndrome. Natural Treatment For Autism, Dyspraxia, Dyslexia, ADD/ADHD, Depression And Schizophrenia.* 2004. Medinform Publishing.
2. Cooper FA. *Cholesterol And The French Paradox.* 2006. Zeus Publications.
3. Enig MG. *Know Your Fats: The Complete Primer For Understanding The Nutrition Of Fats, Oils, And Cholesterol.* Bethesda Press, Silver Spring, MD, 2000.
4. Epstein SS. *Unreasonable Risk.* 2001. Published by Environmental Toxicology, PO Box 11170, Chicago, USA.
5. Fallon S, Enig M. *Nourishing Traditions. The Cookbook That Challenges Politically Correct Nutrition And The Diet Dictocrats.* 1999. New Trends Publishing, Washington DC 20007.
6. Graveline D. *Lipitor – Thief Of Memory, Statin Drugs And The Misguided War On Cholesterol.* Infinity Publishing, Haverford, Pennsylvania.
7. Graveline D. *Statin Drugs Side Effects.* 2007. www.spacedoc.net
8. Kaayla T Daniel. *The Whole Soy Story: The Dark Side of America's Favourite Health Food.* 2006. New Trends Publishing.
9. Kauffman JM. Malignant Medical Myths. 2006. Infinity Pub.
10. Ravnskov U. *The Cholesterol Myths. Exposing The Fallacy That Saturated Fat And Cholesterol Cause Heart Disease.* 2000. New Trends Publishing.
11. Rogers S. *Tired Or Toxic? A Blueprint For Health.* 1990. Prestige Publishers.
12. Sandor Ellix Katz. *Wild Fermentation.* 2003. Chelsea Green Publishing.
13. Schapiro Mark. *Exposed. The Toxic Chemistry Of Everyday Products And What's At Stake For American Power.* Chelsea Green Publishing.
14. Weston A Price. *Nutrition And Physical Degeneration.* 1939. New Trends Publishing.

www.thincs.org – a website for *Cholesterol Sceptics*, a non-commercial organisation of doctors and scientists, who oppose the prevalent dogma about cholesterol and heart disease.

www.westonaprice.org – a website for *The Weston A. Price Foundation,* a charity founded in 1999, dedicated to restoring traditional nutrient-dense foods to the western diet through education and research.

www.chelseagreen.com – a website for Chelsea Green Publishing, who publish books about healthy food, sustainable organic farming, protecting the planet and environment, and sustainable living.

Index

Reviews

"Another vintage Dr Campbell-McBride book – controversial in its take on natural fats, but refreshing in her candid, no-nonsense style and approach to much needed lifestyle and dietary modifications."

Kenneth Bock, M.D., FAAFP, FACN, CNS
Author of the book " Healing the New Childhood Epidemics:
Autism, ADHD, Asthma, and Allergies"

The history of medicine is rife with practices that actually increased suffering and shortened life, such as bloodletting and treatment with mercury compounds. But nothing compares in detrimental effects to the unscientific cholesterol theory of heart disease, now being used to justify lowfat, low-cholesterol diets for the whole population. The theory is so blatantly wrong that a whole crop of literature has appeared to chronicle its faults. But unlike most of the debunkers offering alternative theories on the cause of heart disease, only Dr. Natasha Campbell-McBride zeros in on the most likely cause—the devitalized, additive-laden modern diet, especially the toxic processed vegetable oils that have replaced nutritious animal fats. *Put Your Heart in Your Mouth!* provides not only a well-written, easy-to-understand expose, but also a practical plan for preventing heart disease and regaining health, one that involves a return to traditional foods and an avoidance of environmental pollutants and common household chemicals. And her recipe section is fantastic! *Put Your Heart in Your Mouth!* is must reading for anyone interested in diet and health.

Sally Fallon, President
The Weston A. Price Foundation
Author of the book "Nourishing Traditions"

It has been my pleasure to read this book. The style of writing is both pleasing and easy to understand. Its organization is appropriate to the stated goal of keeping your body healthy. I particularly like the statement, "If your body fails you where will you live?" Dr Campbell-McBride has blended an abundance of information from the cause of atherosclerosis to a delightful assortment of old country recipes in such a manner that every word seems appropriate and flows evenly. And she even found room towards the end to seriously trounce the powers that be for getting us into our present nutritional mess. Obviously we cannot trust our leaders. After 40 years of anti-cholesterol brain-washing I have become thoroughly disenchanted with our leadership. I raised my family on the low cholesterol/low fat diet and counseled all my patients to do the same. I talked at professional organzations and classrooms of the dangers of whole milk, eggs and butter and have written thousands of prescriptions for what choles-terol buster was in vogue at the time. It is terribly difficult to know that because I followed national guidance, I was wrong all that time. Now I am angry at those who guided me and determined it shall not happen again. I thank you for this book and its cutting edge information

Duane Graveline MD. MPH, former NASA astronaut, aerospace medical research scientist, flight surgeon and family doctor. Author of the books "Statin Drugs Side Effects" and "Lipitor, Thief of Memory"